the Abs Diet
Eat Right Every Time Guide

DAVID ZINCZENKO
Editor-in-Chief of Men'sHealth.
Author of the *New York Times* bestseller *The Abs Diet*
WITH TED SPIKER

RODALE

Notice

Distributed to the trade by Holtzbrinck Publishers

ISBN-13 978–1–59486–238–0 paperback
ISBN-10 1–59486–238–9 paperback

4   6   8   10   9   7   5   paperback

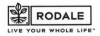

We inspire and enable people to improve their lives and the world around them
For more of our products visit **rodalestore.com** or call 800-848-4735

Contents

Acknowledgments

SEEING THE ABS DIET come to fruition has been one of the great pleasures of my life. Seeing it make a real impact on the lives of tens of thousands of Americans has been one of the great rewards. For all of it, I have to thank a number of extraordinarily talented, hard-working, and dedicated people who continue to support, encourage and inspire me. In particular:

Steve Murphy, whose courage and commitment to editorial quality has made Rodale Inc. the best publishing company in the world to work for.

The Rodale family, without whom none of this would be possible.

Jeremy Katz, executive editor of *Men's Health* Books, whose wisdom and guidance has made The Abs Diet into an extraordinary success.

Ben Roter, whom I want to be when I grow up.

Steve Perrine, who can make a silk purse out of just about anything.

The entire *Men's Health* editorial staff, the smartest and hardest-working group of writers, editors, researchers, designers, and photo directors in the industry. Most important, a big shout out to Chris Krogermeier, Marilyn Hauptly, Jennifer Giandomenico, Erin Hobday, Phillip Rhodes, Brenda Miller, and everyone else who worked so hard and so fast to publish this book in record time.

My brother, Eric, whose relentless teasing shamed me into taking better care of myself. (Dude, you are sooo dead. . . .)

My mother, Janice, who raised two of us nearly single-handedly. Your strength and kindness guide my every action.

My dad, Bohdan, who left this world way to early. I wish you were still here.

Elaine Kaufman, who still lets me order off the menu.

And special thanks also to: Mary Ann Bekkedahl, Michael Bruno, Jeff Csatari, Aimee Geller, Karen Mazzotta, Jon Hammond, Cathy Gruhn, Joe Heroun, Samantha Irwin, George Karabotsos, Charlene Lutz, Patrick McMullan, Peter Moore, Jeff Morgan, Myatt Murphy, Megan Phillips, Scott Quill, Cindy Ratzlaff, Leslie Schneider, Joyce Shirer, Bill Stump, Sara Vigneri, Bug and Fester, and my stepmother, Mickey.

And to Rose. On the rollercoaster of life, you've taught me to let go of the safety bar and reach my hands into the air.

INTRODUCTION

Eat Right Every Time
The Abs Diet Way to a Flat Belly

DIET IS A FOUR-LETTER word.

That may sound like a strange sentence with which to start a diet book. But then again, this is no ordinary diet book.

We think of a diet as something we "go on." A high school reunion looms, or a family vacation to beach territory is planned, or some other event that tells us it's time to bear down and get rid of that extra layer of flab comes up. And so we do—we "go on" a diet. Then, once we've lost the desired weight, we "go off" the diet and go back to our habits of eating cold macaroni and cheese while standing over the kitchen sink. Soon enough, another important event looms, and we're back on another diet again. Up and down, up and down goes our weight, but mostly, over time, it goes up. That's because deprivation diets and fads like eating low-fat, eating low-carb, or eating nothing but grapefruit just don't work in the long run. In fact, they stress your body so much that your body responds by trying even harder to store fat, especially in the midsection.

A recent study in the *American Journal of Preventive Medicine* found that about 60 percent of Americans who try to lose weight do so by restricting their calorie intakes, with roughly one in 10 skipping meals in a desperate attempt to strip off the pounds. But study after study has shown that yo-yo dieting is one of the best ways to ensure your belly will get bigger and flabbier in the months and years ahead.

Well, those days are over!

The Abs Diet is a revolutionary new way of eating, one that's swept America in the last year and helped tens of thousands of people lose hundreds of thousands of pounds. In fact, with the Abs Diet—a simple, six-times-a-day eating plan that will never let you get hungry—you can lose 10, 15, even 20 pounds, from your belly first, in 6 weeks or less.

The Abs Diet isn't a traditional diet, because you'll eat so much delicious food—from steak to strawberries, bread to bacon, soup to nuts—that you'll never want or need to stray from it. In fact, if you're ever hungry on the Abs Diet—well, then, you're not on the Abs Diet.

See, I know how hard it is to lose weight using traditional methods. As a boy growing up in small-town Pennsylvania, I too struggled with a weight problem. I made bad choices—choosing fast food over smart food, then trying to starve myself to get my body in the shape I wanted it. Sure enough, I'd get hungry, and there I'd be, barking my lunch order into a clown's mouth once again. My brother, Eric, used to invite his friends over to watch my dietary indiscretions: "Don't disturb the big animal," he'd tell his buddies. "It's feeding."

But all that's changed. As the editor-in-chief of *Men's Health*, I've spent the past 10 years poring over cutting-edge research in nutrition, fitness, weight loss, and exercise. And what I've learned, I've distilled into the Abs Diet—a program that's been proven time and time again to strip away belly fat and leave you looking and feeling better than ever.

The Secret to Perfect Weight Control Is in Your Hands

THE ABS DIET REVOLVES around a dozen delicious, convenient foods I call the ABS DIET POWER 12. All you need to do is eat the acronym: **A**lmonds and other nuts, **B**eans and other legumes, **S**pinach and other green vegetables, **D**airy (low-fat), **I**nstant oatmeal, **E**ggs, **T**urkey and other lean meats, **P**eanut butter, **O**live oil, **W**hole-grain breads and cereals, **E**xtra-protein (whey) powder, **R**aspberries and other berries.

Yup, you read that right: You get to eat healthy protein, healthy fats, healthy carbs—there's hardly anything you need to give up on this program. Ice cream? Sure. Grilled cheese sandwiches? Yup. Uncle Frank's famous chili? You bet. All I want you to do is eat more good food, more often, and to toy with the ingredients of your favorites to make them just as delicious—and twice as nutritious. And as for the few foods I do want you to say goodbye to—anything that stains your fingers orange, for example—well, I've come up with some great, tasty, healthful alternatives.

The Abs Diet is so easy even Jessica Simpson could handle it. (And she'd get to eat Chicken of the Sea even if it really was chicken!) There's no measuring, no counting calories, no complicated equations, no hours-in-the-kitchen recipes. Just simple, smart, delicious food you'll enjoy all day long.

But even though the Abs Diet is simple, modern life is complicated. The grocery stores and chain restaurants are filled with foods that look healthy but really aren't; foods that are packed with high-calorie sweeteners that actually increase your appetite; foods that are greased up with unhealthy, chemically altered fats that clog up your plumbing; and foods that have had all their nutritional value stripped from them before they're wrapped in cellophane and set on the supermarket shelf. And even family life comes fraught with its own perils: In a survey of 274 single and married women by Texas Tech University Health Sciences Center, researchers found that almost 60 percent of married women were obese, compared to just 43 percent of singles. "Women in larger households have four times the odds of being obese in comparison to women who live alone," says study author James E. Rohrer, Ph.D. He suggests that more people in the household translates into more food in the fridge and a risk of obesity that is four times greater than that of women who live solo.

And that's why I've created this sequel—*The Abs Diet Eat Right Every Time Guide*—to help you make smart, healthy choices on the fly, whether you're cooking up the family dinner or ordering out on a romantic date. Wherever you may be, *The Abs Diet Eat Right Every Time Guide* will show you how to eat more of the great foods out there and teach you to avoid the fat bombs that are looking to spoil your waistline.

Our relationship with food is a complicated one, especially in America, the land of plenty. Sixty-five percent of American adults are obese or overweight, and for good reason: We've become a country that considers drive-throughs fine dining, that saves money if we order two pizzas instead of one, that loves bosses who treat the office to doughnuts, that's been snowed into thinking sausage is a diet food, and that builds its food pyramids with an order of 50 wings.

With *The Abs Diet Eat Right Every Time Guide*, you'll be armed—literally, to the teeth—with the information you need to make the right choices. From Arby's to Zabar's, I've listed the best foods to buy—and the worst foods to avoid—in every shopping and dining situation. Slip this book inside your jacket pocket or into your purse and be ready whenever, wherever hunger strikes.

Stay Lean—Not Hungry

I TRUST THAT if you've read this far, you're inspired by the idea that you can rebuild your body. But every person who wants to lose fat is motivated by different factors—whether it's because you want to feel better, live longer, look better in a bathing suit, run faster, or avoid having your kids mistake you for a Sea World attraction. No matter your motivation, I think building a diet plan that works into your lifestyle is the most important element for success.

Like I said at the beginning of this book, diet is a four-letter word. It's been twisted around to mean eating less, not eating more or eating better. Say the word and all you see is a 6-month stint of celery sticks and rice cakes. Well, wrong. You should stop thinking about "dieting" and start thinking about building a healthy "eating plan." Even the people you'll read about in this book—people who have lost more than 20 pounds in 6 weeks—found themselves forgetting about the word *diet*.

Take Jon Armond, who traded in his beer gut for a flat one with a 35-pound weight loss in 9 weeks. Jon says he doesn't even miss the foods he used to eat.

"I found myself not even consumed with dieting," Jon says. "I've never been on a diet where you didn't have to think about being on the diet all the time." (See his story on page 76.) That's because the Abs Diet is a system that's easy to follow because it never leaves you hungry and gives you the nutritional balance to have all of your cravings fulfilled.

Eat More—and Weigh Less!

MOST DIETS ARE ABOUT losing—losing meals, losing muscle mass, losing energy. The Abs Diet is about gaining—gaining health and fitness, gaining time and energy, gaining delicious foods you can eat whenever you want. Just look at all you have to gain:

A longer life! Belly fat is the most dangerous kind of fat. That's because belly fat often comprises both subcutaneous fat (fat that's under your skin) and visceral fat (fat that lies beneath your stomach muscles, snug up against your internal organs). It's this second type, visceral fat, which can cause you some long-term harm.

Here's why: In a lean, healthy person, the liver uses both fat and glycogen (i.e., blood sugar) as energy. But if your belly is hard to the touch and protrudes out in front of you, it means your liver is basically encased in a layer of fat. With so much fat on hand, your liver gets lazy, forgets about glycogen, and just burns fat for energy. Now, normally, burning fat is good—but not without glycogen to balance it. Your liver is like a big iron stove in your living room. You can fill it with clean, dry wood—that's the glycogen. Or you can fill it with rotten fruit, egg shells, and styrofoam containers—that's the fat. Both will burn, but one will burn cleanly, and the other will create a horrible, stinky mess.

In your body, that horrible stinky mess is excess cholesterol—the byproduct of a liver that burns more fat than glycogen. Perhaps even worse, once your liver gets used to burning fat, it forgets how to properly manage blood sugar. In one report, researchers concluded that visceral fat is the single-best predictor of diabetes. So factor in the higher cholesterol, the increased risk of diabetes, and all the complications of the two, and you realize that losing that fat is just as important to your long-term health as losing that eyebrow ring is to your future employment. But that's really only the beginning of the story. Shedding fat from your frame is essential to living long and healthy. Consider:

▶ A Canadian study of 8,000 people found that those with the weakest abdominal muscles (an indicator for fattier abdominal regions) had twice the death rate of those with stronger ones.

▶ Many studies show that men with waists larger than about 35 inches have an increased risk of heart disease.

▶ A Swedish study found that cancer rates are 33 percent higher in obese patients than in lean ones.

▶ Overweight men are 50 percent more likely to develop heart diseases, 360 percent more likely to develop diabetes, and 16 percent more likely to die of a first heart attack.

Bottom line: Lose fat, gain years. You don't have to be George Steinbrenner to know who gets the better end of that trade.

More and better sex! Sure, losing weight can turn you from a clown to a Clooney, from a Jujube to an Angelina Jolie. But besides the side effects of looking and feeling better (which gives you more confidence and makes you more attractive to others), losing fat helps with the mechanics of sex. Being overweight makes you 50 percent more likely to have erectile dysfunction. Of course, there are many factors that control sexual dysfunction in both men and women, but one of the major ones is a supply-and-demand issue. See, when you're sexually excited, your brain sends an all-points bulletin to your pants. *Wet bathing suit ahead, prepare for engagement.* With that message, your brain sends blood downward to cause an erection in a man or stimulate arousal-sensing and lubricating organs in a woman. But when you're overweight, the aftereffects of the afternoon's burrito supreme gum up your blood vessels and thus narrow the arteries that lead to Shangri La. Without a sufficient blood supply, nothing happens. If there's no gas in the tank, your car ain't going anywhere.

A pain-free and injury-proof life! While the core goal of this book is to help you decipher the tricky menu mines you'll encounter through life, another important part of the Abs Diet is transforming your body with a modest amount of exercise. That will teach your body to grow and maintain lean muscle mass. I'll review the workout principles briefly in Chapter 11, but as part

of the plan, you'll be doing some work to strengthen your abdominal region. That is, you'll teach your abdominal muscles to be
strong. That's not just so you can score a modeling contract.
That's because strong abdominal muscles are the infrastructure
of your body. Your abs play a role in just about every physical
movement you make. They help you run, lift, have sex, stretch,
bend, pick up your kids, and shimmy through clothes racks. But
most important, they act—along with your lower back—as your
internal girdle to support you through the everyday rigors of life.
One U.S. Army study showed that those people with the strong-
est abdominal muscles were the least likely to be injured (for all
kinds of injuries, not just lower-back ones), and that points to
the crucial role that strong abdominal muscles play. Strong
abdominal muscles will help prevent and alleviate back pain—
one of the most debilitating and most common injuries for both
men and women.

It helps to realize that abdominal muscles don't really work in
isolation; they work as a cohesive group that crisscrosses your
midsection and attaches to your spine. When abdominal muscles
are weak, other muscles in your body have to pick up the slack.
They end up overcompensating, and they end up causing back
pain and strain or even more serious back problems.

Abs! If you haven't figured it by now, Sherlock, then let me
explain: This program is about living a healthier life. It'll help
you lose weight, it'll help you gain control of what you eat, and
it'll help turn your body into a fat-burning, muscle-building jug-
gernaut. Ultimately, this book is about striving to meet your
individual goals and looking the way you want to look, and that's
where the abs come in. Abs are the byproduct of your new out-
look on eating and exercising. They're the reward for following a
plan that makes you healthier. Of course, if you're one bonbon
away from a total couch collapse, it's going to take you a little
longer than someone who's only 5, 10, or even 20 pounds over

their ideal weight. (The typical standard for men is that you need to have a body-fat percentage of around 10 percent to have visible abs. For women, it's around 14 percent.) The fact is, everyone has abs, and everyone has the potential to see their abs. It's just a matter of banishing the fat off your gut so you can. Surely, some people are blessed with high-quality genetics, metabolism, or lipo docs, but the potential is there for everyone.

Turn Fat into Muscle!

MOST DIET PLANS DEPEND on willpower for success. The Abs Diet, on the other hand, recruits an often untapped but highly potent ally in your search for slim—your own body!

See, one of the most potent fat-burners around is lurking right below your own skin. It's muscle, and building more can turn your body into a fat-burning machine. For each pound of muscle you build, you'll burn an extra 50 calories a day—just sitting still. If you were to build just 10 pounds of new muscle, you'd burn off enough extra calories to drop 50 pounds of fat in 1 year—again, simply by sitting still.

Of course, you can't build that muscle by sitting still. So I've included in this book a super-simple workout built around an easy weight-training program that anyone can do. It won't turn you into a gym rat, the Incredible Hulk, or the governor of California. But it will help you trade flab for lean, sexy muscle. (Feeling eager? Turn to page 173 for a quick peek at the Abs Diet Workout.)

Take Back Control of Your Body— And Your Life!

YOU DON'T HAVE TO just take my word for it. Listen to other people who've embraced the Abs Diet—people like Linda Toomey, who lost 20 pounds in 6 weeks, while caring for four small children; or Jim Phillips, who was stuck in a weight rut for years until he found this revolutionary and easy plan; or Kyle Snay, who lost more than 20 pounds on the program and alleviated all of his back pain while doing so. As of now, there are more than 100,000 people taking the Abs Diet Challenge (you can find it on www.absdiet.com). The stories of the many people who have tried and succeeded on the Abs Diet show the power of the plan.

Now, with *The Abs Diet Eat Right Every Time Guide*, you have a passport to success no matter where you and your stomach may wander. What I want is for you to use the Abs Diet Powerfoods as the guiding philosophy for the way you eat. With more than 100 recipes in this book, you'll cook up plenty of tasty ways to help you lose fat. But I also want you to use this guide to help you manage situations when you face more tough questions than Michael Jackson's publicist. It's one thing to eat right when you prepare the foods yourself; it's quite another when you're at the mercy of lard-slinging chefs.

Above all—and this is really the foundation for *Eat Right Every Time*—I want you to feel one way while taking part in the Abs Diet: Satisfied.

Satisfied . . . that you'll never be hungry.

Satisfied . . . that you won't be denied great-tasting foods.

Satisfied . . . that you have the flexibility to eat according to your lifestyle.

Satisfied . . . that you'll have the knowledge to eat right anywhere you go.

Satisfied . . . that the only new pants you'll ever have to buy will be smaller.

Satisfied—make that ecstatic—with your new body!

THE ABS DIET
CHEAT SHEET

THIS AT-A-GLANCE GUIDE summarizes the principles of the Abs Diet: the 6-week plan to flatten your stomach and keep you lean for life.

SUBJECT	GUIDELINE
Number of meals	Six a day, spaced relatively evenly throughout the day. Eat snacks 2 hours before larger meals.
The **ABS DIET POWER 12**	Base most of your meals on these 12 groups of foods. Every meal should have at least two foods from the list.
	Almonds and other nuts **B**eans and legumes **S**pinach and other green vegetables
	Dairy (fat-free or low-fat milk, yogurt, cheese) **I**nstant oatmeal (unsweetened, unflavored) **E**ggs **T**urkey and other lean meats
	Peanut butter **O**live oil **W**hole-grain breads and cereals **E**xtra-protein (whey) powder **R**aspberries and other berries
Portion size	While many diets center around controlling portion size, the Abs Diet is designed to be self-controlling. The high-fiber, high-protein foods you'll encounter in this book will fill you up and keep you feeling full for hours. Your body will tell you when it's time to eat—and when it's time to stop.

SUBJECT	GUIDELINE
Secret weapons	Each of the ABS DIET POWER 12 has been chosen in part for its stealthy, healthy secret weapons—the nutrients that will help power up your natural fat burners, protect you from illness and injury, and keep you lean and fit for life!
Nutritional ingredients to emphasize	Protein, monounsaturated and polyunsaturated fats, fiber, calcium.
Nutritional ingredients to limit	Refined carbohydrates (or carbs with high glycemic index), saturated fats, trans fats, high-fructose corn syrup.
Alcohol	Limit yourself to two or three drinks per week, to maximize the benefits of the Abs Diet plan.
Ultimate Powerfood	Smoothies. The combination of the calcium and protein in milk, yogurt, and whey powder, combined with the fiber in oatmeal and fruit, makes them one of the more filling and easy options.
Cheating	One meal a week, eat anything you want.
Exercise program	Optional for the first 2 weeks. Weeks 3 through 6 incorporate a 20-minute, full-body workout 3 days a week. Emphasis is on strength training, brisk walking, and some abdominal work.
At-home workout	Gym workouts and at-home workouts are both detailed to excuse-proof your fitness plan.
Abdominal workout	At the beginning of two of your strength-training workouts. One exercise for each of the five different parts of your abs.

ABS DIET SUCCESS STORY

INSPIRED TO LOSE, INSPIRED TO WIN

Name: Bret Freeman

Age: 38

Height: 5'10"

Weight, Week 1: 205

Weight, Week 6: 183

Weight, Week 17: 175

"I was just basically tired of being a fat slob," says Bret Freeman, who had been a lean, fit wrestler in high school but steadily gained weight over the years.

"I tried Atkins and all the fad diets out there. I'd go on and off, and it always seemed like I gained back more weight than what I started out with," says Freeman, who once reached an all-time high of 245 pounds. "I tried The Zone diet, and that thing was so dang complicated; you had to put so much thought into what you ate, good sugars and bad sugars, what it did to your insulin levels. It was horrible."

When Freeman heard about how simple the Abs Diet was, he couldn't wait to get started. So he ordered it, read it through in a day and a half and started the following Monday. At the same time, he bought a home gym and started the exercise program. The pounds started coming off immediately.

"I think the Abs Diet worked for me for a combination of reasons, but one was that it kept me eating delicious food all day long," he says. "People would notice how much weight I lost, and they'd say, 'You must be starving yourself.' And I'd tell them, 'You wouldn't believe how much I eat.' "

The change? Besides the pounds, Freeman lost inches. He started the diet in snug 38s, and now his 32s are a little loose. "I think I'm ready to go down to a 30." Motivated by Lance Armstrong's story, he's now set to do a couple triathlons, and he's been asked to be the head coach for the high school junior varsity wrestling team. Plus, there's the added satisfaction he feels when he goes to his sons' football games, where he hasn't seen other parents since last season. Freeman says, "One friend joked that they saw my wife, and they thought she got a new husband because I looked so different."

And in a way, she did.

Chapter I

YOUR WEIGHT IS
REALLY NOT YOUR
FAULT

EVERYONE HAS ENEMIES. Batman has the Joker. Duke has UNC. Joan Rivers has gravity. You? Sure, your cranky neighbor may slice your perennials when he mows the lawn, and the boss's henchman may boil your blood, but to me, the biggest enemies you face are the profiteering junk-food merchants of the food industry.

In a time-strapped society and in your time-strapped life, these piranhas prey on consumers who need a quick fix—a quick fix of fat, fries, and foods designed to hypnotize you with their taste and stretch you at your waist. As you surely can see at any interstate exit, mall food court, or stretch of commercialized suburbia, we live in a world of fast food. We have a world rich with hot dog vendors, pizza windows, order-at-the-counter restaurants, chain restaurants, and extra-value meals—a world where, even when you want to eat healthy, it sometimes feels impossible to do so. These places pelt you with chips, suffocate your innards with ice cream, and shoot rapid-fire Goobers straight into your mouth.

But fast food doesn't need to be fat food. Convenient eating doesn't have to mean that fat conveniently claims squatter's rights on your gut. Easy eating doesn't mean greasy eating.

The secret of the Abs Diet's success is that you can follow it no matter where you are. If you just remember to eat the acronym—the ABS DIET POWER 12—you'll stay lean, fit, and healthy no matter where you are. You don't have to fall victim to kitchens that have more grease than a mechanic's fingernails, and you don't have to stop enjoying the taste of food to do so.

You can eat fast.

You can enjoy what you eat.

And you can be free from hunger, deprivation, and culinary boredom.

I want to arm you with the information you need to make smart decisions about eating on the fly or on a Friday family night out. Before I explain the Abs Diet plan and give you hundreds of choices for what to eat no matter what situation you're in, it's important to review your nutritional friends and enemies. You know, there are only a few things that you can do to fundamentally change the way your body's chemicals, hormones, and organs function, but the one major thing that you do that changes your body's internal systems is eat. Ultimately, your health is dictated by the nutrients that travel through your bloodstream once they pass through your Fritos hole. Here's a quick primer on the pitfalls of your nutritional world.

Your Enemies

The Hunger-Booster: High-Fructose Corn Syrup (HFCS)

I believe there's one primary reason why many people fail on diets—and why they eat poorly to begin with. They're so damn hungry.

Sound simple? Anatomically, it's a little more complicated. And the complication has come in the form of a little-known but shockingly ubiquitous food additive called High-Fructose Corn Syrup (HFCS).

Never heard of HFCS before? Then you'll be even more shocked by this next fact: You, the average American, consume almost 63 pounds of it each year.

Sit and think about that for a moment. Sixty-two pounds of it each year—or about 228 extra calories every day—and you don't even know what it is.

And you're not going to be any happier once you find out: See, up until the 1970s, most sweets were made with simple white sugar. Bad for you, but it was what it was. You sated your sweet tooth, your body absorbed the calories, and you got full pretty fast. But about 3 decades ago, food manufacturers discovered an easier way to make sodas, cereals, yogurts, and some 40,000 more manufactured foods taste sweeter. They developed HFCS, which is derived from corn and is many times cheaper—and sweeter—than simple sugar. Today, HFCS is added to a shocking number of foods, including foods you wouldn't equate with sweeteners: ketchup, pasta sauce, and even crackers. And it's screwing up America's metabolic system.

Mechanically, the system works like this: When you eat any type of carbohydrate (like bread or fruit), your body releases insulin to regulate your body weight—pushing those carb calories into your muscles to be used as energy or storing them for later use. Then, like a shut-off mechanism on a gas pump, it suppresses your appetite. That's the signal that tells your body to stop filling; your tank is full.

The problem is that fructose doesn't stimulate insulin so your body doesn't register it the way it registers simple white sugar. That's why it's possible to see people drink 2-liter bottles of soft drinks in a single sitting. Thirty years ago, that would have been an impossible task, but today, HFCS makes the same number of calories go down and, incredibly, still leaves you hungry for more.

Your muscles still need energy, so you crave more food and more sweets. And so you eat more foods containing HFCS, and the cycle continues. Less energy, more flab. HFCS could well stand for Here's Flab Coming to your Stomach.

You don't need to eliminate this artificial foodstuff from your diet entirely, but you need to ensure your meals don't revolve around it, as many Americans' do. So start checking the food labels: If HFCS is listed first or second on the ingredient list, look at the chart on the nutrition label to see how much sugar the food contains. If it's just a gram or two, it's fine. But if you see a food that has 8 or more grams of sugar, and HFCS is prominent on the list of ingredients, it's a sign that you should leave it on the shelf.

FOODS HIGH IN HFCS OR FRUCTOSE	REPLACE WITH
Regular soft drinks	Unsweetened sparkling water or diet soda
Commercial candy (such as jelly beans)	Chocolate candy (check the label; some chocolate bars have HFCS)
Pancake syrup	Real maple syrup
Frozen yogurt	Ice cream
Fruit-flavored yogurt	Artificially sweetened or sugar-sweetened yogurt
Highly sweetened cereals	Sugar-free or low-sugar cereals
Pasta sauce	Sugar-free pasta sauce

The Artery Hardener: Trans Fat

If HFCS is Bonnie, then trans fat is Clyde, because together, the duo is responsible for some seriously heinous crimes against your body.

First, it's important to know that dietary fats are a little like college bands, minus the long hair and low pants. Some are actually good, and some are unbelievably bad. Trans fats falls into the latter category. Trans fat increases the amount of bad cholesterol in your body, for example, and has been linked to an increased risk of heart disease, diabetes, and a weakened immune system.

Scientists have estimated that trans fat contributes to more than 30,000 premature deaths every year.

So what exactly is this stuff? Once again, it's a Frankenstein monster that's come lumbering out of the labs of the food industry.

Trans fat is created by combining vegetable oil (a liquid) with hydrogen to create partially hydrogenated oil, or trans fatty acids. Once infused with hydrogen, liquid vegetable oil turns into a solid at room temperature, becoming what we recognize today as Crisco or margarine.

Trans fats are beloved by the food and restaurant industries for several reasons. Number one, they're cheap. Number two, they can stick around seemingly forever without going bad. (How gross is that?) Number three, you can add them to myriad foods in a way you can't add regular oil—a cookie with vegetable oil in it will ooze all over the supermarket shelf, but one with partially hydrogenated oil in it will stay crisp and tantalizing. So it's no surprise that food marketers, eager to deliver the sensuous flavor and mouth feel of fat to millions of unsuspecting consumers, now add partially hydrogenated oils to all sorts of things—chips, frozen foods, fries, muffins, to name a few.

But think about what trans fats are: Fats that are supposed to be liquid but are turned into solids. Now think about what they do when they get inside you. Instead of melting like they would in their natural state, they try to revert to their waxy, solid nature. Once you understand that heart disease and stroke are caused in part by waxy buildups of fat solids in the circulatory system, it's easy to put two and two together. Turning oils into solids isn't doing us a favor—not by a long run.

The good news is that the U.S. government is finally recognizing the dangers of trans fats. In 2003, food companies were required to list these trans fats for the first time. At least this gives you the power to see the enemy you need to fight (though food companies have several years to phase the new nutritional labels in). In the meantime, use these tactics to reduce your intake of trans fats:

▶ Check the ingredient list for "hydrogenated" or "partially hydrogenated." The higher these ingredients are on the label, the more trans fats they contain (with the exception of processed peanut butter, which contains trace amounts).

▶ Decode the food label. For those products that don't list trans fats, add all the fat grams together that are listed on the label and then subtract that number from the total fat content. The number you're left with is the estimate for the amount of trans fat.

▶ Snack on baked chips or chips fried in peanut oil instead of ones with vegetable shortening (check the ingredient list).

▶ Pick high-protein breakfasts like eggs or Canadian bacon instead of waffles. If you have toast, use jelly instead of margarine.

▶ At a restaurant, ask what kind of oil the chef uses. You want to hear olive oil—not shortening.

▶ When eating dinner out, avoid bread, which may be filled with trans fats. It's better to pick a baked potato, soup, or a salad.

▶ Blot oil from your fries as quickly as possible. A napkin can absorb excess grease.

IF YOU WANT	PICK THIS TRANS FAT-FREE OPTION
Candy bar	Dove dark chocolate bar
Cereal	Kellogg's Frosted Mini-Wheats or Post Premium Raisin Bran
Cookies	Archway fat-free cookies or Pamela's Products gourmet cookies
Crackers	Ryvita Multigrain crackers
French fries	McCain 5-Minute Shoestring French Fries
Potato chips	Ruffles Natural sea-salted, reduced-fat chips

The Belly Buster: Saturated Fats

Just the name sounds threatening, doesn't it? Saturated fats, as in they're going to sink into your stomach and saturate your organs with soft little globs of putty. Bleeech!

And the truth is just as gross as you imagine it to be. Your body likes to burn some kinds of fats—polyunsaturated (from vegetables) and monounsaturated (from nuts and seeds) fats—as energy. But your body would rather save saturated fats around your belly to use for future energy in case, I dunno, your plane crashes in the jungles of the Philippines or something. Assuming there's no Battan Death March in your immediate future, however, your body will continue to hold onto the fat it's stored, and the more you eat, the more you wear. Besides raising cholesterol rates, saturated fats have also been shown to increase your risk for heart disease and some types of cancer.

Saturated fats are found primarily in meats and dairy products. "But wait!" you say. "Aren't meats and dairy products part of the ABS DIET POWER 12?" Yes, and that's why I emphasize lean meats like turkey, chicken, fish, and some cuts of beef and recommend that you look for low-fat dairy products like low-fat milk or low-fat yogurt whenever possible. The trick is to get the most nutrients—muscle-building protein and fat-fighting calcium—with the least amount of saturated fats.

The Energy Sucker: Refined Carbohydrates

Consider the simple wheat stalk: There it stands, soaking up the sun and minding its own business, a single droplet in a vast sea of amber waves. Who'd have thought this humble grain would spark a controversy more complicated than the JFK assassination? And yet, the dietary landscape is wrought by forces arguing grain's place at the American dinner table. On this side, the USDA food guide pyramid, which calls for six to eleven servings of grains a day. And on that side, the Atkins addicts and other no-carb adherents who believe that simple stalk of wheat is evil incarnate.

The truth is . . . well, the truth is in neither corner, but somewhere more towards the middle.

The truth is that the human body can't survive without carbohydrates, because grains—like fruits, vegetables, and other carbs—provide crucial energy to feed the brain, the muscles, and

HOW METABOLISM WORKS—AND HOW TO MAKE IT WORK FOR YOU

Even if you're lying in bed, lounging on the couch, or sitting on the toilet as you're reading this, your body is burning calories. It's burning calories to keep your heart beating, your lungs breathing, your brain dreaming about Cabo San Lucas. . . . Hey, wake up!

That calorie burn I'm referring to is your metabolism, and how high it's revving is what determines whether you're losing fat right now—or gaining it. See, your body burns calories all the time, and it burns them in three different ways. One, you burn them when you eat, simply through the act of digestion (remember, it takes more energy to digest protein than it does carbs). Two, you burn calories by exercise and movement, whether you're running a marathon or just walking down the hall. And the last way you burn calories is when you're at rest; that's called your *basal metabolism*, and it refers to the way your body uses fuel when you're not doing anything. Incredibly enough, this is when the majority of your calories are burned—while you're doing nothing.

That explains, in part, why watching those calories tick away on the treadmill or the exercise bike is an exercise in frustration. If the majority of calories are burned during your non-exercising times, then it makes sense to boost your calorie burn during those times, and the way you do that is by adding muscle. In fact, for every pound of muscle you build, your body will need to burn off up to 50 extra calories a day, just sitting around doing nothing. Add 6 pounds of muscle, and you're burning up to 300 extra calories a day, just hanging out being you.

Later on in this book, I'll walk you through the basics of the Abs Diet Workout, a muscle-building, fat-burning, 20-minute workout that will help you create the body you've always wanted.

the metabolism. Grains also provide crucial vitamins, minerals, and fiber, all of which the body needs to stay healthy. For example, a recent study at Brigham and Women's Hospital found that women who consumed 800 or more micrograms of folate a day had 29 percent less risk of high blood pressure than those who consumed less than 200 micrograms daily. Folate is just one of the many nutrients found in carbohydrates.

But the anti-carb movement does have its points to make, because most of the carbohydrates in the American diet aren't rich in all those great nutrients and fiber. They're "refined carbohydrates," such as white sugar, white bread, bagels, waffles, et cetera. Most baked goods, in fact, are made from grains that have had all their great nutrients "refined" out of them.

This causes serious dietary problems for the carb lover. A slice of bread made with whole grains—wheat, oats, or what have you— is full of fiber. Fiber expands once it's in the belly, taking up space, slowing the digestive process, and keeping your energy and hunger levels even for several hours. Take out the fiber, though, and those carb calories go shooting through the digestive track faster than Bill Clinton at a sorority party. There's a rush of blood sugar as the carbs are quickly digested, a burst of energy, and then a letdown as insulin stores the blood sugar and your body cries out for more.

That's why the ABS DIET POWER 12 includes whole-grain breads and cereals, along with fruit, vegetables, and other carbohydrate sources. Carbs have the energy you need; you just have to choose wisely. Read the label; you want to see the words "whole grain" on your bread, cereal, and cracker boxes whenever possible.

Your Friends

The Muscle Builder: Protein

You may think of protein as the staple ingredient for bodybuilders or the Atkins crowd, but protein has more super powers than the

Hall of Justice. For one, protein helps kick-start your metabolism. It takes your body twice as much energy to break down protein as it does to break down carbohydrates, so when you eat a high-protein meal, you actually burn off additional calories at the dinner table. In one study, for example, people who ate a high-protein diet burned more than twice as many calories in the hours after their meals as people on a high-carbohydrate diet.

Protein also flips your satisfaction switch. When you start your meal with protein—say, downing a glass of fat-free milk before breakfast or ordering the shrimp cocktail appetizer at dinner—your body registers its satiation level earlier on, and you wind up eating less. And that effect can carry on throughout the day. Some studies have shown that, if all calories are equal, people who eat a high-protein meal feel fuller and eat less at their next meal than those who don't. In another study, subjects who followed a high-protein diet lost an average of 20 pounds each, compared to just 11 pounds lost by participants who followed a low-protein diet. Amazingly, protein not only burned away fat, it burned away belly fat. The high-protein dieters lost twice as much abdominal fat as their low-protein dieting counterparts.

The Cholesterol Cutters: Polyunsaturated and Monounsaturated Fats

Ten years ago, if I had told you to eat more fat, I'd have been dragged from my office by the diet police and run out of town on a rail. Although it's generally a good idea to cut down on some kinds of fats—like trans fats and saturated fats—other kinds are actually good for you. Good? Heck, they're great.

Our bodies need fat. We need it to deliver vitamins throughout our bodies. We need it to produce testosterone—the hormone that leads to muscle growth. And we need it to keep satiated and full. In fact, one of the important things we've learned recently is that reducing your fat intake doesn't necessarily decrease your body-fat percentage over the long haul. In a recent study at Brigham and Women's Hospital in Boston, participants were put on either a low-fat or moderate-fat diet. After 6 months, the two groups lost about the same amount of weight. But when doctors checked in after 12 months, they discovered that the low-fat eaters had not only gained back what they lost, but they had added an average of 6 pounds! The dieters who were allowed to eat fats, however, lost an average of 9 pounds—and kept it off.

So, as the song goes, Grease is the Word—as long as it's the

ABS DIET SUCCESS STORY

SHE HAD THE GUTS TO LOSE HERS

Name: Linda Toomey

Age: 35

Height: 5'4"

Weight, Week 1: 145

Weight, Week 6: 126

Body-Fat Percentage, Week 1: 36

Body-Fat Percentage, Week 6: 25

When Linda Toomey had her fourth baby, she knew that she had to get the weight off. She was still carrying an extra 20 pounds she'd gained from her third child, and she wanted to act quickly, because she knew the longer she waited, the harder it would be. At 145 pounds and with four children under the age of 6, she knew that her own health—and belly—might take a backseat to everything else going on in her life. "I'm the queen of excuses," she says.

Toomey also knew that she needed as much energy as possible—especially considering she wasn't getting a full night's sleep anyway, caring for a newborn.

right kind of grease. The two kinds of fats that you'll incorporate into your eating plan are polyunsaturated and monounsaturated. Polyunsaturated fats include the famous omega-3's, which are found in fish like salmon and tuna and work to help clear your arteries. But more research shows that polyunsaturated fat also plays a role in helping speed your metabolism. Studies have shown that people who take omega-3's burned more calories throughout the day than those who don't. And a recent study of more than 35,000 women discovered that those who ate fish high

"At night, I expected to be tired," she says. "But I was tired 2 hours after I woke up."

Her goals: Get her body back, have more energy, and strengthen her back to be able to meet the demands of carrying larger-than-average children.

"I tried other diets, but being so crazy and busy, I didn't have a lot of time for exercise or food preparation. I needed something that was easy and fast to prepare," Toomey says.

She found it in the Abs Diet. "It's not really a diet," she says. "It's a life-long eating plan. I think knowing that you can eat carbs and not resist cravings was one of the key factors. The eating plan was extremely easy to follow, and the whole family could enjoy the meals. I didn't have to prepare different foods for myself."

Toomey also included the 20-minute exercise plan and strengthened her abdominals and lower back to the point where she has no problem lifting her children.

In 6 weeks, Toomey dropped 19 pounds and went from 35-percent body fat to 25. And she also went from a size 14 dress to size 6.

"I'm hoping it motivates a lot of women," Toomey says. "In the past after being pregnant, the waist was extremely hard for me. I may have lost inches from everywhere else in the past, but the waist was my real difficult area. It's amazing how it progressed in a short time."

in omega-3's had the lowest body mass indexes (BMIs)—even lower than vegetarians. (And if you're a vegetarian, there's still no excuse: Flaxseed and flaxseed oil are also loaded with omega-3's, and you can find them in a health food store. Get the ground flaxseed so you can toss it on cereal or into smoothies.)

The other kind of good fat—monounsaturated—is found in nuts, olives, avocados, and olive and canola oils. Monounsaturated fats reduce cholesterol levels, as well, and they also help burn fat and keep you satiated. One study found that subjects who ate a meal with oil high in monounsaturated fats felt fuller than those who ate one cooked with the polyunsaturated kind. And that's a primary approach to how you need to eat: Balance your foods with the ingredients that keep your hunger in check. You want to keep your stomach satisfied—not the folks at Big & Tall.

The Appetite Suppressor: Fiber-Rich Carbohydrates

As I stated earlier in this chapter, it's not the "carbohydrate" part you should be concerned about, it's the "fiber" part. Whole-grain breads and cereals, oatmeal, and berries—these are the real weapons of mass destruction, and the mass they seek to destroy is the one collecting around your waist.

There are two types of fiber: soluble and insoluble. Let's see if I can define them both in one paragraph without making you nod off.

Soluble fiber, like the kind you find in oatmeal, apples, and other fruits and grains, likes to hang out in your stomach. While it's hanging out, it does two things. First, it slows digestion, giving you longer-burning energy throughout the day. Second, it bonds with digestive acids, which happen to be made from cholesterol. When fiber splits, it takes the digestive acids with it, forcing your body to pull cholesterol from your bloodstream to make more. Presto, your cholesterol profile improves. Insoluble fiber, meanwhile, does not like to hang around. It shoots through your plumbing like Drāno, picking up miscellaneous fats and whatever else happens to be loitering in your system and ushering them out the back. So both types of fiber help keep all your pipes and fittings in order, and if you eat them regularly, they should delay any need for professional plumbing services in the near future.

The Weight-Loss Wonder: Calcium

In the past few years, researchers have begun studying the effects of calcium-rich dairy foods on weight management. And quite frankly, it's hard not to be cowed by the evidence.

For example, researchers at Harvard Medical School showed that those who ate three servings of dairy a day—to total the recommended 1,200 milligrams of calcium daily—were 60 percent less likely to be overweight. But some of the most exciting research came from a study in which researchers put subjects on diets that were 500 calories a day less than what they were used to eating. The subjects lost weight—about a pound of fat a week. But when researchers put another set of subjects on the same diet but added dairy to their meals, their fat loss doubled, to 2 pounds a week. Same calorie intake, double the fat loss. Calcium, it seems, is going to be one of the most exciting new areas of research about weight loss and metabolism, and that's why it's an important part of the ABS DIET POWER 12.

Chapter 2

NEVER GO HUNGRY AGAIN

The ABS DIET POWER 12

THE GOVERNMENT USES acronyms: FBI, CIA, DOT. Media corporations use acronyms: ABC, CNN, BET. We love acronyms because they're easy to remember. (Do you even recall what CNN stands for after all these years?)

The Abs Diet comes with its own acronym—the ABS DIET POWER 12. They are 12 foods you want to look for and fit into your eating plan whenever you can.

I don't know about you, but if I had to consult a chart, formulate some kind of substitution plan, or calculate calories at every turn, I'd starve. Eating plans need to be simple, because life is complicated. And that's what the ABS DIET POWER 12 is—simple. Figuratively, it stands for the principles of what this body-transforming diet is all about. Literally, it stands for:

Almonds and other nuts
Beans and legumes
Spinach and other green vegetables

Dairy (fat-free or low-fat milk, yogurt, cheese)
Instant oatmeal (unsweetened, unflavored)
Eggs
Turkey and other lean meats

Peanut butter
Olive oil
Whole-grain breads and cereals
Extra-protein (whey) powder
Raspberries and other berries

As you can see, these 12 foods, or food groups, if you will, constitute a veritable cornucopia of dietary choices. You can use the acronym when you're shopping, when you're cooking at home, and when you're eating out.

The crux of the diet and *The Abs Diet Eat Right Every Time Guide* is that if you can revolve your meals around these 12 Powerfoods, you'll know exactly what to order, what to shop for, and how to eat right every time. You'll have armed yourself with the "friend" category of nutrients that will help your body lose fat and gain lean muscle, and you'll have shunned the "enemy" category of junk foods that threaten to lay waste to your waist. Here's a quick overview of the ABS DIET POWER 12 and what they have to offer.

How to read the key: For at-a-glance scanning, I've included the following icons under the descriptions of each of the Abs Diet Powerfoods. Each icon demonstrates which important roles each food can help play in maintaining optimum health.

Builds muscle: Foods rich in muscle-building plant and animal proteins qualify for this seal of approval, as do foods rich in certain minerals linked to proper muscle maintenance, such as magnesium.

Helps prevent weight gain: Foods high in calcium and fiber (both of which protect against obesity) as well as foods that help build fat-busting muscle tissue earn this badge of respect.

Strengthens bone: Calcium and vitamin D are the most important bone builders, and they protect the body against osteoporosis. But beware: High levels of sodium can leach calcium out of bone tissue. Fortunately, all of the Powerfoods are naturally low in sodium.

Lowers blood pressure: Any food that's not high in sodium can help lower blood pressure—and earn this designation—if it has beneficial amounts of potassium, magnesium, or calcium.

Fights cancer: Research has shown that there is a lower risk of some types of cancer among people who maintain low-fat, high-fiber diets. You can also help foil cancer by eating foods that are high in calcium, beta-carotene, or vitamin C. In addition, all cruciferous (cabbage-type) and allium (onion-type) vegetables get the cancer protection symbol because research has shown they help prevent certain kinds of cancer.

Improves immune function: Vitamins A, E, B_6, and C; folate; and the mineral zinc help to increase the body's immunity to certain types of disease. This icon indicates a Powerfood with high levels of one or more of these nutrients.

Fights heart disease: Artery-clogging cholesterol can lead to trouble if you eat foods that are predominant in saturated and trans fats, while foods that are high in monounsaturated or polyunsaturated fats will actually help protect your heart by keeping your cholesterol levels in check.

#1: Almonds and Other Nuts

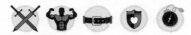

Superpowers: builds muscle, fights cravings

Secret weapons: protein, monounsaturated fats, vitamin E, fiber, magnesium, folate (peanuts), phosphorus

Fights against: obesity, heart disease, muscle loss, wrinkles, cancer, high blood pressure

Sidekicks: flaxseed, pumpkin seeds, sunflower seeds, avocados

Imposters: salted or smoked nuts

These days, you hear about good fats and bad fats the way you hear about good cops and bad cops. One's on your side, and one's gonna beat you silly. Oreos fall into the latter category, but nuts are clearly out to help you. They contain the monounsaturated fats that clear your arteries and help you feel full.

All nuts are high in protein and monounsaturated fat. But almonds are like Jack Nicholson in *One Flew over the Cuckoo's Nest*: They're the king of the nuts. A handful of almonds provides half the amount of vitamin E you need in a day and 8 percent of the calcium. Almonds also contain 19 percent of your daily requirement of magnesium—a key component for muscle building. In a Western Washington University study, people taking extra magnesium were able to lift 20 percent more weight and build more muscle than those who weren't. Eat as much as two handfuls of almonds a day. A Toronto University study found that men can eat this amount daily without gaining any extra weight. A Purdue University study showed that people who ate nuts high in monounsaturated fat felt full an hour and a half longer than those who ate fat-free food (rice cakes, in this instance). If you eat 2 ounces of almonds (about 24 of them), it should be enough to suppress your appetite—especially if you wash them down with

8 ounces of water. The fluid helps expand the fiber in the nuts to help you feel fuller. Also, eat almonds with the nuts' nutrient-rich skins on them.

Here are ways to seamlessly introduce almonds and other nuts into your diet.

▶ Add chopped nuts to plain peanut butter.

▶ Toss a handful of nuts on cereal, yogurt, or ice cream.

SUPPLEMENT SMARTS

You can get nearly every nutrient in the ABS DIET POWER 12 from a bottle or a can. Health food stores are filled with multivitamins and dietary supplements that promise better health and nutrition. But I want you to be eating real, wholesome, delicious foods, not popping pills.

One main reason—besides the fact that eating your meals in pill form makes you feel like you're on the set of *Logan's Run*—is that fruits, vegetables, whole grains and other Powerfoods offer not only the aforementioned vitamins, minerals, and fiber, but hundreds of "micronutrients," as well. These micronutrients—many of which are only now being studied and classified—may have tremendous protective properties that scientists are still trying to discover. So the more real food you eat, the more real nutrition you get.

That said, there are two nutrients that aren't readily available through traditional food sources. If you want to supplement your healthy diet with some extra weight-loss power, consider:

▶ Conjugated linoleic acid (CLA) is a fatty acid that's been shown to aid in weight loss. Researchers recently reported that subjects taking CLA for 1 year lost up to 8.7 percent of their body fat. The recommended dosage is 3 grams daily.

▶ Pyruvate is an antioxidant that may help aid weight loss, as well. In two trials, people taking pyruvate in addition to a low-fat diet stepped up their weight loss. The recommended dosage is 25 grams daily.

▶ Put almond slivers in an omelet.

▶ For a quick popcorn alternative, spray a handful of almonds with nonstick cooking spray and bake at 400 degrees for 5 to 10 minutes. Take them out of the oven and sprinkle them with a mixture of either brown sugar and cinnamon or cayenne pepper and thyme.

One caveat, before you get all nutty: Smoked and salted nuts don't make the cut here, because of their high sodium content. High sodium can mean high blood pressure.

Although it's not technically a nut, I want you to consider adding ground flaxseed to your food. As I pointed out earlier, 1 tablespoon contains only 60 calories, but it packs in omega-3 fatty acids and has nearly 4 grams of fiber. It has a nutty flavor, so you can sprinkle it into a lot of different recipes, add some to your meat or beans, spoon it over cereal, or add a tablespoon to a smoothie.

#2: Beans and Legumes

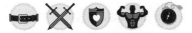

Superpowers: builds muscle, helps burn fat, regulates digestion

Secret weapons: fiber, protein, iron, folate

Fights against: obesity, colon cancer, heart disease, high blood pressure

Sidekicks: lentils, peas, bean dips, hummus, edamame

Imposters: refried beans, which are high in saturated fats; baked beans, which are high in sugar

Most of us can trace our resistance to beans to some unfortunately timed intestinal upheaval (third-grade math class, a first date gone awry). But beans are, as the song says, good for your heart; the more you eat them, the more you'll be able to control your hunger. Black, lima, pinto, garbanzo—you pick the bean (as long as it's not refried—refried beans are loaded with fat). Beans are a low-calorie food packed with protein, fiber, and iron—ingredients crucial for building muscle and losing weight. Gastrointestinal disadvantages notwithstanding, beans serve as one of the key members of the Abs Diet cabinet because of all their nutritional power. In fact, you can swap in a bean-heavy dish for a meat-heavy dish a couple of times per week; you'll be lopping a lot of saturated fat out of your diet and replacing it with higher amounts of fiber.

The best beans for your diet are:

▶ Soybeans

▶ Pinto beans

▶ Chickpeas (garbanzo beans)

▶ Navy beans

▶ Black beans

▶ White beans

▶ Kidney beans

▶ Lima beans

#3: Spinach and Other Green Vegetables

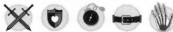

Superpowers: neutralizes free radicals, which are molecules that accelerate the aging process

Secret weapons: vitamins including A, C, and K; folate; minerals including calcium and magnesium; fiber; beta-carotene

Fights against: cancer, heart disease, stroke, obesity, osteoporosis

Sidekicks: cruciferous vegetables like broccoli and brussels sprouts; green, yellow, red, and orange vegetables like asparagus, yellow beans, and peppers

Imposters: none, as long as you don't fry them or smother them in fatty cheeses

You know vegetables are packed with important nutrients, but they're also a critical part of your body-changing diet. I like spinach in particular because one serving supplies nearly a full day's worth of vitamin A and half of your vitamin C. It's also loaded with folate—a vitamin that protects against heart disease, stroke, and colon cancer. To incorporate spinach into your diet, you can take the fresh stuff and use it as lettuce on a sandwich or try stir-frying it with a little fresh olive oil and garlic.

Another potent power vegetable is broccoli. It's high in fiber and more densely packed with vitamins and minerals than almost any other food. For instance, broccoli contains nearly 90 percent of the vitamin C of fresh orange juice and almost half as much calcium as milk. It is also a powerful defender against diseases like cancer because it increases the enzymes that help detoxify carcinogens. Tip: With broccoli, you can skip the stalks. The florets have three times as much beta-carotene as the stems, and they're also a great source of other antioxidants. Sauté olive oil and garlic and douse them with hot sauce.

If you hate vegetables, you can learn to hide them but still reap the benefits. Try pureeing them and adding them to marinara sauce or chili. The more you chop and puree vegetables, the more invisible they become, and the easier it is for your body to absorb them.

#4: Dairy (Fat-Free or Low-Fat Milk, Yogurt, Cheese)

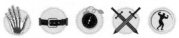

Superpowers: builds strong bones, fires up weight loss

Secret weapons: calcium, vitamins A and B_{12}, riboflavin, phosphorus, potassium

Fights against: osteoporosis, obesity, high blood pressure, cancer

Sidekicks: cottage cheese, low-fat sour cream

Imposters: whole milk, frozen yogurt

Dairy is nutrition's version of a typecast actor. It gets so much attention for one thing it does well—strengthening bones—that it gets little or no attention for all the other stuff it does well. It's about time for dairy to accept a breakout role as a vehicle for weight loss. Just take a look at the mounting evidence: A University of Tennessee study found that dieters who consumed between 1,200 and 1,300 milligrams of calcium a day lost nearly twice as much weight as dieters getting less calcium. In a Purdue University study of 54 people, those who took in 1,000 milligrams of calcium a day (about 3 cups of fat-free milk) gained less weight over 2 years than those with low-calcium diets. Researchers think that calcium probably prevents weight gain by increasing the breakdown of body fat and hampering its formation. Low-fat yogurt, cheeses, and other dairy products can play an important role in your diet. But as your major source of calcium, I recommend milk for one primary reason: volume. Liquids can take up valuable room in your stomach and send the signal to your brain that you're full. Adding in a sprinkle of chocolate powder can also help curb sweet cravings while still providing nutritional power.

#5: Instant Oatmeal (Unsweetened, Unflavored)

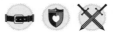

Superpowers: boosts energy and sex drive, reduces cholesterol, maintains blood sugar levels

Secret weapons: complex carbohydrates and fiber

Fights against: heart disease, diabetes, colon cancer, obesity

Sidekicks: high-fiber cereals like All-Bran and Fiber One

Imposters: cereals with added sugar and high-fructose corn syrup

Oatmeal is the Bo Derek of your pantry: It's a perfect 10. You can eat it at breakfast to propel you through sluggish mornings, a couple of hours before a workout to feel fully energized by the time you hit the weights, or at night to avoid a late-night binge. I recommend instant oatmeal for its convenience. But I want you to buy the unsweetened, unflavored variety and use other Powerfoods such as milk and berries to enhance the taste. Preflavored oatmeal often comes loaded with sugar calories.

Oatmeal contains soluble fiber, meaning that it attracts fluid and stays in your stomach longer than insoluble fiber (like vegetables). Soluble fiber is thought to reduce blood cholesterol by binding with digestive acids made from cholesterol and sending them out of your body. When this happens, your liver has to pull cholesterol from your blood to make more digestive acids, and your bad cholesterol levels drop.

Trust me: You need more fiber, both soluble and insoluble. Doctors recommend we get between 25 and 35 grams of fiber per day, but most of us get half that. Fiber is like a bouncer for your body, kicking out troublemakers and showing them the door. Fiber protects you from heart disease, and it also protects you from colon cancer by sweeping carcinogens out of the intestines quickly.

A Penn State study also showed that oatmeal sustains your blood sugar levels longer than many other foods, which keeps your insulin levels stable and ensures you won't be ravenous for the few hours that follow. That's good, because spikes in the production of insulin slow your metabolism and send a signal to the body that it's time to start storing fat. Since oatmeal breaks down slowly in the stomach, it causes less of a spike in insulin levels than foods like bagels. Include oatmeal in a smoothie or as your breakfast.

(A U.S. Navy study showed that simply eating breakfast raised metabolism by 10 percent.)

Another cool fact about oatmeal: Preliminary studies indicate that oatmeal raises the levels of free testosterone in your body, enhancing your body's ability to build muscle and burn fat and boosting your sex drive.

#6: Eggs

Superpowers: builds muscle, burns fat

Secret weapons: protein, vitamin B_{12}, vitamin A

Fights against: obesity

Sidekicks: none

Imposters: none

For a long time, eggs were considered pure evil, and doctors were more likely to recommend tossing eggs at passing cars than into omelet pans. That's because just two eggs contain enough cholesterol to put you over your daily recommended value. Though you can cut out some of the cholesterol by removing part of the yolk and using the whites, more and more research shows that eating an egg or two a day will not raise your cholesterol levels, as once previously believed. In fact, we've learned that most blood cholesterol is made by the body from dietary fat, not dietary cholesterol. And that's why you should take advantage of eggs and their powerful makeup of protein.

The protein found in eggs has the highest "biological value" of protein—a measure of how well it supports your body's protein need—of any food. In other words, the protein in eggs is more effective in building muscle than protein from other sources, even milk and beef. Eggs also contain vitamin B_{12}, which is necessary for fat breakdown.

#7: Turkey and Other Lean Meats

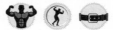

Superpowers: builds muscle, improves the immune system

Secret weapons: protein, iron, zinc, creatine (beef), omega-3 fatty acids (fish), vitamins B_6 (chicken and fish) and B_{12}, phosphorus, potassium

Fights against: obesity, various diseases

Sidekicks: shellfish, Canadian bacon

Imposters: sausage, bacon, cured meats, ham, fatty cuts of steak like T-bone and rib-eye

A classic muscle-building nutrient, protein is the base of any solid diet plan. You already know that it takes more energy for your body to digest the protein in meat than it does to digest carbohydrates or fat, so the more protein you eat, the more calories you burn. Many studies support the notion that high-protein diets promote weight loss. In one study, researchers in Denmark found that men who substituted protein for 20 percent of their carbs were able to increase their metabolism and increase the number of calories they burned every day by up to 5 percent.

Among meats, turkey is a rare bird. Turkey breast is one of the leanest meats you'll find, and it packs nearly one-third of your daily requirements of niacin and vitamin B_6. Dark meat, if you prefer, has lots of zinc and iron. One caution, though: If you're roasting a whole turkey for a family feast, avoid self-basting birds, which have been injected with fat.

Beef is another classic muscle-building protein. It's the top food source for creatine—the substance your body uses when you lift weights. Beef does have a downside; it contains saturated fats, but some cuts have more than others. Look for rounds or loins (that's code for extra-lean); sirloins and New York strips are less fatty than prime ribs and T-bones. Wash down that steak with a glass of fat-free milk. Research shows that calcium (that magic bullet again!) may reduce the amount of saturated fat your body absorbs. Choose cuts on the left side of the chart below. They contain less fat but still pack high amounts of protein.

LEAN BEEF (55 calories and 2–3 grams of fat per 1-ounce serving)	MEDIUM-FAT BEEF (75 calories and 5 grams of fat per 1-ounce serving)
Flank steak	Corned beef
Ground beef (extra-lean or lean)	Ground beef (not marked as lean or extra-lean)
London broil	
Roast beef	Prime cut
Tenderloin	

To cut down on saturated fats even more, concentrate on fish like tuna and salmon, because they contain a healthy dose of omega-3 fatty acids as well as protein. Those fatty acids lower levels of a hormone called leptin in your body. Several recent studies suggest that leptin directly influences your metabolism: The higher your leptin levels, the more readily your body stores calories as fat. Researchers at the University of Wisconsin found that mice with low leptin levels have faster metabolisms and are able to burn fat faster than animals with higher leptin levels. Mayo Clinic researchers studying the diets of two African tribes found that the tribe that ate fish frequently had leptin levels nearly five times lower than the tribe that primarily ate vegetables. A bonus benefit: Researchers in Stockholm studied the diets of more than 6,000 men and found that those who ate no fish had three times the risk of prostate cancer than those who ate it regularly. It's the omega-3's that inhibit prostate cancer growth.

#8: Peanut Butter

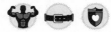

Superpowers: boosts testosterone, builds muscle, burns fat

Secret weapons: protein, monounsaturated fat, vitamin E, niacin, magnesium

Fights against: obesity, muscle loss, wrinkles, cardiovascular disease

Sidekicks: cashew and almond butters

Imposters: mass-produced sugary and trans fatty peanut butters

Yes, PB has its disadvantages: It's high in calories, and it doesn't go over well when you order it in four-star restaurants. But it's packed with those heart-healthy monounsaturated fats that can increase your body's production of testosterone, which can help your muscles grow and your fat melt. In one 18-month experiment, people who integrated peanut butter into their diets maintained weight loss better than those on low-fat plans. A recent study from the University of Illinois showed that diners who had monounsaturated fats before a meal (in this case, it was olive oil) ate 25 percent fewer calories during that meal than those who didn't.

Practically speaking, PB also works because it's a quick and versatile snack, and it tastes good. Since a diet that includes an indulgence like peanut butter doesn't leave you feeling deprived, it's easier to follow and won't make you fall prey to other cravings. Use it on an apple, on the go, or to add flavor to potentially bland smoothies. Two caveats: You can't gorge on it because of its fat content; limit yourself to about 3 tablespoons per day. And you should look for all-natural peanut butter, not the mass-produced brands that have added sugar and trans fat.

#9: Olive Oil

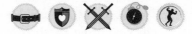

Superpowers: lowers cholesterol and boosts the immune system

Secret weapons: monounsaturated fat, vitamin E

Fights against: obesity, cancer, heart disease, high blood pressure

Sidekicks: canola oil, peanut oil, sesame oil

Imposters: vegetable and hydrogenated vegetable oils, trans fatty acids, margarine

You read extensive information on the value of high-quality fats like olive oil in Chapter 1. But it's worth reiterating here: Olive oil and its brethren will help you eat less by controlling your food cravings; they'll also help you burn fat and keep your cholesterol in check. Do you need any more reason to pass the bottle?

#10: Whole-Grain Breads and Cereals

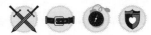

Superpower: prevents your body from storing fat

Secret weapons: fiber, protein, thiamin, riboflavin, niacin, pyridoxine, vitamin E, magnesium, zinc, potassium, iron, calcium

Fights against: obesity, cancer, high blood pressure, heart disease

Sidekicks: brown rice, whole-wheat pastas, whole-wheat pretzels

Imposters: processed bakery products like white bread, bagels, and doughnuts; breads labeled wheat instead of whole wheat

There's only so long a person can survive on an all-protein diet or an all-salad diet or an all-anything diet. You will crave carbohydrates because your body needs carbohydrates. The key is to eat the ones that have been the least processed—carbs that still have all their heart-healthy, belly-busting fiber intact.

Grains like wheat, corn, oats, barley, and rye are seeds that come from grasses, and they're broken into three parts—the germ, the bran, and the endosperm. Think of a kernel of corn. The biggest part of the kernel—the part that blows up when you make popcorn—is the endosperm. Nutritionally it's pretty much a big dud. It contains starch, a little protein, and some B vitamins. The germ is the smallest part of the grain; in the corn kernel, it's that little white seedlike thing. But while it's small, it packs the most nutritional power. It contains protein, oils, and the B vitamins thiamin, riboflavin, niacin, and pyridoxine. It also has vitamin E and the minerals magnesium, zinc, potassium, and iron. The bran is the third part of the grain and the part where all the fiber is stored. It's a coating around the endosperm that contains B vitamins, zinc, calcium, potassium, magnesium, and other minerals.

So what's the point of this little biology lesson? Well, get this: When food manufacturers process and refine grains, guess which two parts get tossed out? Yup, the bran, where all the fiber and minerals are, and the germ, where all the protein and vitamins are. And what they keep—the nutritionally bankrupt endosperm (that is, starch)— gets made into pasta, bagels, white bread, white rice, and just about every other wheat product and baked good you'll find. Crazy, right? But if you eat products made with all the parts of the grain—whole-grain bread, whole-grain pasta, long-grain rice—you get all the nutrition that food manufacturers are otherwise trying to cheat you out of.

Whole-grain carbohydrates can play an important role in a healthy lifestyle. In an 11-year study of 16,000 middle-age people, researchers at the University of Minnesota found that consuming three daily servings of whole grains can reduce a person's mortality risk over the course of a decade by 23 percent. (Tell that to your buddy who's eating low-carb.) Whole-grain bread keeps insulin levels low, which keeps you from storing fat. In this diet, it's especially versatile because it'll supplement any kind of meal with little prep time. Toast for breakfast, sandwiches for lunch, bread with a dab of peanut butter for a snack. Don't believe the hype. Carbs—the right kind of carbs—are good for you.

Warning: Food manufacturers are very sneaky. Sometimes, after refining away all the vitamins, fiber, and minerals from wheat, they'll add molasses to the bread, turning it brown, and

CAN YOU STOMACH THIS?

When I tell people about the Abs Diet, I'm often asked about the issue of portion control. In most diets, portion control is a key element, but the Abs Diet comes with its own portion control built in. Because you'll be eating lots of fiber, protein, and healthy fats, the foods you eat on the Abs Diet will fill you up and give you long-running energy, so you won't feel the need to binge and won't have the urge to stuff your stomach like Santa's sack. But just for kicks, let's look at what happens to your body when you do overeat.

▶ Your stomach, which is the size of your closed fist, doesn't crave more servings. When you're full, it is, too.

▶ But if you're eating very quickly—a common problem with junk food—your stomach becomes distended and can swell to as much as three times its original size. It then pushes against your lungs and diaphragm.

▶ If you really overeat, some of the food may not immediately reach your stomach, so it loiters in your esophagus, causing acid-reflux–related belching and nausea.

▶ Your liver works overtime to digest the surplus food by producing excess bile—an emulsifier that helps fats and oils pass through your intestines. Your intestines also crank out extra digestive enzymes.

▶ After all this stressful work, your GI system can't take it and rebels. Your body looks for a way to dump the excess cargo— by any means necessary.

put it on the grocery shelf with a label that says wheat bread. It's a trick! Truly nutritious breads and other products will say whole-wheat or whole-grain. Don't be fooled.

#11: Extra-Protein (Whey) Powder

Superpowers: builds muscle, burns fat

Secret weapons: protein, cysteine, glutathione

Fights against: obesity

Sidekick: ricotta cheese

Imposter: soy protein

Protein powder? What the heck is that? It's the only Abs Diet Powerfood that you may not be able to find at the supermarket, but it's the one that's worth the trip to a health food store. I'm talking about powdered whey protein, a type of animal protein that packs a muscle-building wallop. If you add whey powder to your meal—in a smoothie, for instance—you may very well have created the most powerful fat-burning meal possible. Whey protein is a high-quality protein that contains essential amino acids that build muscle and burn fat. But it's especially effective because it has the highest amount of protein for the fewest number of calories, making it fat's kryptonite. Smoothies with some whey powder can be most effective before a workout. A 2001 study at the University of Texas found that lifters who drank a shake containing amino acids and carbohydrates before working out increased their protein synthesis (their ability to build muscle) more than lifters who drank the same shake after exercising. Since exercise increases bloodflow to tissues, the theory goes that having whey protein in your system when you work out may lead to a greater uptake of amino acids—the building blocks of muscle—in your muscle.

But that's not all. Whey protein can help protect your body from prostate cancer. Whey is a good source of cysteine, which your body uses to build a prostate cancer–fighting antioxidant called glutathione. Adding just a small amount may increase glutathione levels in your body by up to 60 percent.

By the way, the one great source of whey protein in your supermarket is ricotta cheese. Unlike other cheeses, which are made from milk curd, ricotta is made from whey—a good reason to visit your local Italian eatery.

#12: Raspberries and Other Berries

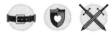

Superpowers: protects your heart; enhances eyesight; improves balance, coordination, and short-term memory; prevents cravings

Secret weapons: antioxidants, fiber, vitamin C, tannins (cranberries)

Fights against: heart disease, cancer, obesity

Sidekicks: most other fruits, especially apples and grapefruit

Imposters: jellies, most of which eliminate fiber and add sugar

Depending on your taste, any berry will do (except Crunch Berries). I like raspberries as much for their power as for their taste. They carry powerful levels of antioxidants, all-purpose compounds that help your body fight heart disease and cancer. the berries' flavonoids may also help your eyesight, balance, coordination, and short-term memory. One cup of raspberries packs 6 grams of fiber and more than half of your daily requirement of vitamin C.

Blueberries are also loaded with the soluble fiber that, like oatmeal, keeps you fuller longer. In fact, they're one of the most healthful foods you can eat. Blueberries beat out 39 other fruits and vegetables in the antioxidant power ratings. (One study also found that rats that ate blueberries were more coordinated and smarter than rats that didn't.)

Strawberries contain another valuable form of fiber called pectin (as do grapefruits, peaches, apples, and oranges). In a study from the *Journal of the American College of Nutrition*, subjects drank plain orange juice or juice spiked with pectin. The people who got the loaded juice felt fuller after drinking it than those who got the juice without the pectin. The difference lasted for an impressive 4 hours.

MIDNIGHT MADNESS

If you're dying for a midnight snack, chances are you're probably more bored, restless, or worried than you are hungry—especially if you've eaten six meals already today. The key here is to do as little harm as possible and to get back to bed. Milk, oatmeal, and bananas contain trace amounts of melatonin, the send-me-to-sleep hormone. Combine them all in one bowl (one instant oatmeal packet made with milk and topped with half a sliced banana) or just have one alone. Backups: A small bowl (½ cup or so) of whole-grain cereal with milk, 2 fig bars, or ¼ cup ice cream.

The Abs Diet Bull's Eye

Variety being the spice of life and all, you're often going to have the opportunity and the desire to mix in foods that don't fall squarely into the ABS DIET POWER 12. That's fine, as long as you keep your eye on the target and try to mix at least two Powerfoods into each meal and snack.

To help keep you focused on the ABS DIET POWER 12, I've created a little game I call the Abs Diet Bull's Eye. In the center of this chart are the foods you want to concentrate on. Around them, in concentric layers, are additional foods you'll no doubt run across every day.

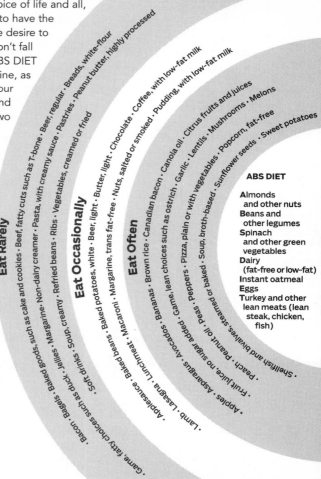

Eat Rarely

Baked goods, such as cake and cookies · Beef, fatty cuts such as T-bone · Beer, regular · Breads, white-flour · Pasta, with creamy sauce · Pastries · Peanut butter, highly processed · Ribs · Vegetables, creamed or fried · Margarine · Non-dairy creamer · Jellies · Soup, creamy · Bacon · Bagels · Baked beans · Baked goods, such as duck ·

Eat Occasionally

Baked potatoes, white · Beer, light · Butter, light · Chocolate · Coffee, with low-fat milk · Nuts, salted or smoked · Pudding, with low-fat milk · Macaroni · Margarine, trans fat-free · Soft drinks · Lunchmeat · Lasagna · Asparagus · Applesauce · Baked beans ·

Eat Often

Bananas · Brown rice · Canadian bacon · Canola oil · Citrus fruits and juices · Garlic · Lentils · Mushrooms · Melons · Game, lean choices such as ostrich · Peppers · Pizza, plain or with vegetables · Popcorn, fat-free · Soup, broth-based · Sunflower seeds · Sweet potatoes · peas · baked · steamed or · Peach · peanut oil · Fruit juice, no sugar added · Avocados · Apples · Shellfish and bivalves ·

ABS DIET

Almonds
 and other nuts
Beans and
 other legumes
Spinach
 and other green
 vegetables
Dairy
 (fat-free or low-fat)
Instant oatmeal
Eggs
Turkey and other
 lean meats (lean
 steak, chicken,
 fish)

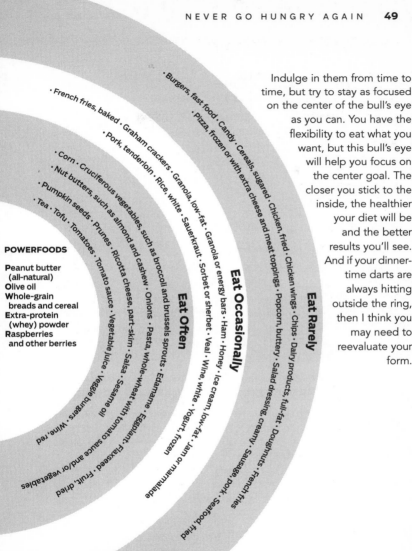

Indulge in them from time to time, but try to stay as focused on the center of the bull's eye as you can. You have the flexibility to eat what you want, but this bull's eye will help you focus on the center goal. The closer you stick to the inside, the healthier your diet will be and the better results you'll see. And if your dinner-time darts are always hitting outside the ring, then I think you may need to reevaluate your form.

POWERFOODS

Peanut butter
 (all-natural)
Olive oil
Whole-grain
 breads and cereal
Extra-protein
 (whey) powder
Raspberries
 and other berries

Eat Often

· Corn · Cruciferous vegetables, such as broccoli and brussels sprouts · Edamame · Eggplant · Flaxseed · Fruit, dried · Nut butters, such as almond and cashew · Onions · Pasta, whole-wheat with tomato sauce and/or vegetables · Pumpkin seeds · Prunes · Ricotta cheese, part-skim · Salsa · Sesame oil · Tea · Tofu · Tomatoes · Tomato sauce · Vegetable juice · Veggie burgers · Wine, red

Eat Occasionally

· French fries, baked · Graham crackers · Granola, low-fat · Granola or energy bars · Ham · Honey · Ice cream, low-fat · Jam or marmalade · Pork, tenderloin · Rice, white · Sauerkraut · Sorbet or sherbet · Veal · Wine, white · Yogurt, frozen

Eat Rarely

· Burgers, fast food · Candy · Cereals, sugared · Chicken, fried · Chicken wings · Chips · Dairy products, full-fat · Doughnuts · French fries · Pizza, frozen or with extra cheese and meat toppings · Popcorn, buttery · Salad dressing, creamy · Sausage, pork · Seafood, fried

HE BEAT THE CURSE
OF THE FAMILY GUT

Name: Jim Phillips

Age: 37

Height: 6'1"

Weight, Week 1: 190

Weight, Week 6: 169

Body-Fat Percentage, Week 1: 24

Body-Fat Percentage, Week 6: 15

Ever since high school, Jim Phillips had been gaining weight—not all at once, but just a few pounds every year. At one point, he found himself at 215 pounds on his 6-foot-1 frame and decided he needed to do something about it. So he took up running, started cutting down on his fat intake, and concentrated on a more vegetarian-like diet. He lost weight and got down to 190. And he stayed at 190—for 5 years. But still, Phillips's gut lingered on.

"I think I kinda wore the weight well, but I knew I was definitely over-weight—even if other people didn't notice it," he says.

One of the places Phillips wore his weight was the infamous Phillips family gut (which he'd inherited through years of soda, pizza, and bagels). After reaching that plateau of 190, Phillips resigned himself to the fact that he was going to stay there, especially as he got older.

Then, he found the Abs Diet.

"As soon as I saw the book, I really liked it because of the approach—telling you the foods to eat, not what you can't," Phillips says. "Psychologically, that was one of the biggest things. I like feeling good about what I'm eating."

Phillips tried the Abs Diet—eating six times a day (up from his habit of light meals early in the day and eating a big dinner) and following an exercise program that emphasizes strength-training and interval-training as the means to burning fat. He really feels that his change in exercise helped him. "I was definitely into a lackadaisical routine the last 4 years. When I changed to a shorter routine and higher intensity, I noticed the difference."

The effect: He dropped 21 pounds in 6 weeks, 9 percentage points off his body-fat percentage, and 4½ inches off his waist. Plus, he has much better energy and fitness levels. Though he ran regularly when he was 190 pounds, he can really feel the difference now. "I never felt as good running as I feel now. My knees aren't hurting. Hills are so much easier. I just did 13 miles yesterday," says Phillips, who has run marathons and is training for another. "Before, I wouldn't have been able to walk the next day after doing that distance. Now it doesn't even bother me."

While he still indulges in an occasional doughnut, he's made a change—for good. "After the fifth or sixth week on the diet, it hit me that I really didn't remember what my old habits were," Phillips says. "The new ways just became natural and something I wanted to live with and how I wanted to eat. It wasn't going to be something I fell off of because I could eat the foods I like to eat."

Chapter 3

THE SIX STEPS TO LIFELONG LEANNESS

Guidelines for Easy Eating

LOTS OF GOOD THINGS come in sixes. Besides the Brady kids and bottles of Bud, there's also that group of muscles that gets title billing on this book. And then there's the Abs Diet guidelines. Six of them. That's it.

It all goes back to the simple principle of, well, simplicity. No matter how nutritionally responsible popular diets are (some are and some aren't, by the way), most of them are more high-maintenance than an old Fiat. They require you to do complicated math, keep dietary journals, or stay "in the zone" (wherever the heck that is). Well, forget that. Instead, I've eliminated all the complex elements and boiled the Abs Diet down to six simple guidelines that don't require a degree in home economics or exotic ingredients you need to order from Madagascar.

What you'll find are that these six general principles aren't really rules; they just serve as the map that shows you the way to your ultimate destination: a lean, strong, and healthy body.

Guideline 1: Eat six meals a day

When people are introduced to the Abs Diet, their first question is this: "How can I lose weight if I'm eating twice as many meals?" The explanation is simple—and delicious.

See, nature doesn't much care if you have abs, which is why Cro Magnon man didn't have buffalo-skin Speedos. Our bodies evolved to do one thing: Stay alive long enough to pass our genes on to the next generation. When our ancestors roamed the jungles and plains, they encountered frequent times of deprivation and hardship. So just like bears in winter, our bodies became adept at storing calories, in the form of fat, to tide us over during times when food was scarce.

The more frequently the body is exposed to times of deprivation, the more it conspires to store fat and to jettison lean muscle tissue. That's because muscle requires more calories to maintain than fat does. The drought hits, the herds move on, and our ancestor starts living on his own muscle tissue. When food returns, his body reacts by bulking up with fat so he can make it through future lean times.

Nowadays, the herd never moves on; it's always there, 24 hours a day, at the drive-through. But people who go on calorie-restrictive diets create a modern version of starvation: They're not eating enough calories to maintain their lean muscle tissue. (In fact, most diets are not fat-loss diets, they're muscle-loss diets.) And as soon as people go off their diets, boom: The body instinctively begins storing fat. It doesn't know that it's being starved on purpose; it only knows it needs to survive the next diet.

But there's more bad news for the starvation-diet set. By burning away muscle, they're sacrificing the body's greatest weapon in the fight against flab. As I said above, muscle requires many more calories to maintain than fat does. In fact, for each pound of muscle you gain, your body burns up to 50 extra calories a day, just sitting still. Now let's say you go on a restrictive diet for a week, and you lose

4 pounds, and half of that is muscle. When you end your diet and return to eating as you normally do, you may be taking in the same number of calories you once did—but your body actually requires 100 calories a day less, because of the muscle you lost. So where do those calories go? Right to your gut. It takes only 3,500 calories to build a pound of fat. So you've now programmed your body to gain a pound

---

ABS DIET SUCCESS STORY

THE ABS DIET HEALS A BAD BACK

Name: Kyle Snay

Age: 36

Height: 6'5"

Weight, Week 1: 227

Weight, Week 6: 205

Weight, Week 9: 199

Kyle Snay knew he needed to get back into shape—fast. Motivation to get in shape came in droves.

Reason 1: His dad. Several years earlier, Snay had made plans to visit his father—whom he didn't know well because his parents had been divorced. But 6 months before Snay was to make his pilgrimage, his dad dropped dead of a heart attack. That's when it hit Snay that his health was something he needed better control of.

Reason 2: His kids. "I was a walking Twinkie for years," Snay says. "When my wife was pregnant with our second child, I said that I really needed to do something to get back in shape at least for my family. I was trying to keep up with our 2 year old, and it was exhausting."

Reason 3: His back. Snay, who's had a herniated disc for 10 years, says, "My big flare-up came when I was bending down to pick up a Doritos chip." After years of twinges, spasms, and pain that laid him up for a couple days at a time, he was told by doctors his choices were surgery or physical therapy.

of fat every 35 days—or more than 10 pounds in the coming year.

Some diet plan, huh?

And yet this is the crux of yo-yo dieting, and it's one of the worst things you can do for your figure and your health. But here's the thing: Most of us go on mini-starvation diets every single day. When we limit ourselves to three meals a day, we're asking our

---

Snay chose neither. He chose the Abs Diet.

After deciding he was going to lose weight, Snay went searching for something hassle-free. "I didn't want to count calories, or carbs, or fat. I read about the Abs Diet in *Men's Health* and noticed results immediately."

Before, Snay never paid attention to what he ate: His staple foods included ice cream and "Oreo soup"—a whole bunch of Oreos in a full bowl of milk. He immediately changed his diet and saw the pounds peel away. Plus, he got a bonus out of it: a better back. "Since I started, I haven't had a twinge, a spasm, or anything—nothing. My back is completely fine," he says. "It's just unreal. That was a huge plus that I wasn't even expecting."

Snay says he really stuck to the principles but appreciates the diet's flexibility. Eating six times a day, he says, makes you feel like you're never really "on a diet."

Now, almost 30 pounds lighter, Snay retrained his metabolism—so much so that he lost his last 5 pounds even when he had to take a week off of exercise and sneak in a few extra cheat meals because he was away at a business conference. He also invents his own recipes following the ABS DIET POWER 12. "I know people who are still trying to do Atkins, and they just pour meat down their stomach. In a couple of weeks, they're still walking around like a bowl of pudding because they're not doing any exercising, and they're taking too many shortcuts," he says.

"I can't ever see myself going back to who I was before," Snay says. "I just can't wait until it gets warm again. I'm going to go out and wash my car—with my shirt off for the first time in years. I'll even stay out there longer and wash my neighbor's car, too."

bodies to operate normally all the time, even though we're inter-
mittently depriving it of fuel, then dumping big heaps of calories
into it every 6 hours or so. That's why eating three squares will
make you round. But if you break those meals into six of them,
you're getting a steady stream of fuel throughout the day to balance what your body is doing.

In fact, the new catchphrase in obesity science is "energy balance." Energy balance refers to taking in throughout the day a
similar number of calories as you're burning off. As long as you're
constantly fueling your body with small meals, you're constantly
teaching it to shed fat. Ideally, you're trying to keep your hourly
calorie surplus or deficit within 300 or 500 calories at all times,
meaning that you're never going long periods without eating, and
you're never overloading your system with too many calories at
one sitting. As you burn calories throughout the day—by exercising, by walking from the parking lot, by jumping up and down
screaming, if that's your thing—the calories you ingest should
stay within similar levels of the calories you burn. That's balance—never having too many calories and never being starved for
more. In one study, researchers gave two sets of dieters the same
daily calorie intake. But one group ate those calories in two big
meals, while the other group ate them in six small meals spread
throughout the day. At the end of the study, those who ate six
meals a day lost an average of 11 pounds in two weeks; those who
ate the same number of calories in just two meals a day also lost
11 pounds, but they lost 3 pounds more of muscle than men eating 6 meals who lost 3 more pounds of fat.

So the Abs Diet works in two ways: By maintaining your energy
balance and by helping you build new muscle. The more lean muscle mass you have, the more energy it takes to fuel it—meaning that
calories go to your muscles to sustain them rather than being con-
verted to fat. That's why I call muscle-building exercise the magic
bullet in the chamber—the secret weapon in your fight against fat.

You'll read much more about the Abs Diet Workout in Chapter 11, and you'll learn how you can build new muscle that jump-starts your metabolism and turns your body into a fat-burning machine. In the meantime, I want you to keep this equation in mind:

MORE FOOD = MORE MUSCLE = LESS FLAB

The alternative:

LESS FOOD = LESS MUSCLE = MORE FLAB

Oh, and one more thing: If you eat six times a day, you never get hungry. If you never get hungry, you never get tired, cranky, or miserable. And if you never get hungry, tired, cranky, or miserable, you never feel the need to drown your hunger pangs or energy drain in a 32-ounce root beer float.

To keep the fat-burners firing, eat your six meals like this:

► Alternate larger meals and smaller ones.

► Eat your snacks roughly 2 hours before lunch, 2 hours before dinner, and roughly 2 hours after dinner.

► Eat to fit your own schedule and lifestyle, but an ideal schedule would look something like this:

8 A.M.: Breakfast
11 A.M.: Snack
1 P.M.: Lunch
4 P.M.: Snack
6 P.M.: Dinner
8 P.M.: Snack

Guideline 2: Revolve your eating around the ABS DIET POWER 12

The ABS DIET POWER 12 is your ticket to eating better anywhere, anytime. While every meal won't consist entirely of Powerfoods, the more Powerfoods you can squeeze into your day, the more quickly and effectively you'll change your body and your life.

For example, let's say you're trapped in some nutritional equivalent of Dante's Inferno, where the only food you have to eat comes out of a vending machine. You could choose the Coke and the tortilla chips (mmm . . . nacho cheese!) and those nifty Dunking Sticks for dessert. Or you could peer through the glass and look for Powerfoods. They're in there . . . the fat-free microwave popcorn, the unsalted peanuts, the low-fat chocolate milk.

Let's see . . . soda, chips, and dunking sticks, or chocolate milk, popcorn, and peanuts. Both sound like junk-food meals, right? So which do you choose? Here's where the magic of the Powerfoods comes into play:

VENDING MACHINE MEAL #1:

Can of Coke 155 calories, 0 g protein, 40 g carbohydrates, 0 g fat, 0 g fiber, 15 mg sodium

1.5-ounce bag of nacho cheese tortilla chips 212 calories, 3 g protein, 27 g carbohydrates, 11 g fat (2 g saturated), 2 g fiber, 301 mg sodium

2 Dunking Sticks 360 calories, 4 g protein, 44 g carbohydrates, 18 g fat (6 g saturated), 1 g fiber, 260 mg sodium

VENDING MACHINE MEAL #2:

8 ounces low-fat chocolate milk 180 calories, 8 g protein, 28 g carbohydrates, 4.5 g fat (3 g saturated), 1 g fiber, 150 mg sodium

94% Fat-free microwave popcorn (3 cups) 120 calories, 4 g protein, 26 g carbohydrates, 2 g fat (0 g saturated), 4 g fiber, 380 mg sodium

1-ounce bag of unsalted peanuts 167 calories, 8 g protein, 5 g carbohydrates, 15 g fat (2 g saturated), 2.5 g fiber, 2 mg sodium

What a difference choosing the Powerfoods can make: Meal #1 has about 50 percent more calories (727 versus 467), and pales in comparison nutritionally to Meal #2. By making your choices based on the Powerfoods, you get three times as much protein, more than twice the fiber, and significantly less fat and sodium.

And that's something you can do no matter where you are,

because every supermarket, every restaurant, every vending machine, and every movie-theater concession stand offers something that contains one or more Powerfoods. And that, my friends, will keep you losing weight—without driving you nuts.

While you're negotiating the nutrition wasteland, I'd like you to keep these three thoughts in mind:

►Incorporate two to three Powerfoods into each of your three major meals and at least one or two of them into each of your three snacks.

►Diversify your food at every meal to make sure you have a combination of protein, carbohydrates, and healthy fat.

►Make sure you sneak a little bit of protein into each snack.

Guideline 3: Drink smoothies regularly

I'll never forget something that one of the first followers of the Abs Diet said. He lost some 20 pounds in the first 6 weeks, and he attributed most of that loss to one part of the diet: the smoothies. It was like getting to go to Dairy Queen every day, he said.

See, smoothies are more than just faux milk shakes packed with healthy ingredients. They're one of the keys to the Abs Diet because they pack your day with more energy than a busload of cheerleaders. In a recent study, researchers found that meal-replacement shakes work brilliantly as a weight-loss method. Subjects who replaced two daily meals with shakes or meal-replacement bars lost about 9 percent of their original body weight.

More important, smoothies feature everything you could possibly want out of a food, like:

►Ease: They take less than 3 minutes to make

►Taste: Like dessert, with one exception. They're guilt-free.

►Satisfaction: Because they're so thick and packed with Powerfoods, they take up valuable room in your stomach to keep you full for hours.

►Effectiveness: With the secret fat-fighter calcium, and satiating fiber and protein, they're some of the most potent meals or snacks you can make.

While Chapter 8 gives you recipes for 27 different kinds of smoothies, I'd also encourage you to mix and match ingredients that fit your tastes. That's the great thing about smoothies. All you have to know is how to open a lid and press a button to make one. So dump in whatever Powerfoods you like, whether it's berries, peanut butter, or oatmeal, and experiment with your own flavors (I advise against the salmon). Then follow these guidelines.

►Drink one or two 8-ounce smoothies a day, as a meal substitute or as a snack. In one study, researchers found that regularly drinking meal replacements increased a man's chance of losing weight and keeping it off for longer than a year.

►Add ice cubes and blend your smoothie for at least 10 minutes. Thicker shakes incorporate a little more air and water but have an increased satiating effect. In one study, researchers found that people stayed fuller longer when they drank thick drinks than when they drank thin ones. Another study found that men who drank yogurt shakes that had been blended until they doubled in volume ate 96 fewer calories a day than men who drank shakes of normal thickness.

►Don't skimp on the yogurt. A University of Tennessee study found that men who added three servings of yogurt a day to their diets lost 61 percent more body fat and 81 percent more stomach fat over 12 weeks than men who didn't eat yogurt. Calcium, baby!

Guideline 4: Stop counting
On the Abs Diet, you'll count the number of pounds you've lost, you'll count the notches on your belt you've gained, you may even

count your lucky stars. But one thing you will not count is calories. Counting calories is for suckers.

For one, most people don't have the time or discipline to record every pretzel stick they eat or weigh the three slices of turkey breast they carved. And two, all calories are not made equally when it comes to metabolism. Instead, the important thing is to eat the right foods. If you do, your body will essentially regulate your caloric intake all by itself. By including a good balance of fiber and protein, you'll be full throughout the day.

What you want to do is think about—not record—the amount of food you eat by sticking to one helping of each food group you eat and keeping the total contents of each meal contained to the diameter of your plate (and please, no high-rise mashed potatoes).

Guideline 5: Watch what you drink

I think a diet with lots of restrictions is like a roller-coaster without hills or a zoo without animals. What's the point of having a diet plan if it's so regimented and boring that nobody's going to be able to follow it? That's why the Abs Diet is about what you can eat, not what you can't. But the one place you really have to be careful is in what you drink.

Alcohol and soda, along with a lot of juice blends and prepackaged iced teas, contain empty, non-nutritious calories that will work against you in pursuit of a better body. While alcohol has some health benefits in moderation, it also encourages you to eat more, slows down fat-burning, and increases fat-storing. Drink water (eight 8-ounce glasses is ideal), diet soda, and low-fat milk. I encourage you to keep the booze in the cooler for the first 6 weeks of the plan, but if you drink, limit yourself to no more than two or three drinks a week.

Guideline 6: Go ahead, cheat

Americans are rebels at heart—inside each of us lies an inner James Dean or Mae West, an Ali or a Madonna, someone who wants to break the rules and make the world march to their own tune. Well, rebellion is built right into the Abs Diet.

On the Abs Diet, I want you to cheat—with one whatever-you-want meal a week. That way, you can satisfy your cravings without derailing your commitment to the ABS DIET POWER 12. Of course, in the Abs Diet, there are enough great variations that you'll probably lose the urge for wings, Oreos, or Oreo-flavored wings pretty quickly. In fact, many people who've used the Abs Diet reported that they didn't even feel the urge to cheat, but they loved the fact that they had it as an option.

Now, if you're going to cheat on me, I want you to do it conscientiously. When considering an adulterous encounter with an unhealthy food bear in mind the following:

▶Plan it. If you schedule your cheat meal, you'll be less likely to eat on impulse at other times during the week. Make it every Friday, when you meet the gang from work for beer and potato skins. Or every Sunday, when you treat yourself to cake and ice cream while watching Mike Wallace mysteriously not age.

▶Really, do it. While you don't have to cheat, it may help you in the long run. Researchers at the National Institutes of Health found that men who ate twice as many calories in a day as normal increased their metabolism by 9 percent in the 24-hour period that followed.

▶Stick to one a week. The cheat meal is like walking on a cliffside trail. It's entirely safe—unless you step over the line. You need to view the cheat meal as satisfaction instead of temptation and remain focused on your weight-loss goals. You'll be better off for it.

Chapter 4

SHOP 'TIL YOU DROP (POUNDS)

The Complete Abs Diet Grocery List

AS FAR AS I'M CONCERNED, every time someone walks into a supermarket, they should play "Welcome to the Jungle" over the loudspeaker. Supermarkets are one of the most confusing and mind-numbing places on earth, right up there with the Balkans and your local DMV. Supermarkets have one goal: to sell you more calories than you actually came in to buy. The easiest foods to find are usually the worst for you (a special on doughnuts!), and in the checkout lane, eight rows of candy taunt you like the hecklers at a Knicks game. There's a reason why they're called supermarkets, you know; they're super marketers.

So next time you go food shopping, you should notice things, like . . . the cracker aisle never moves. Sure, the junk—and it usually is junk—on each aisle's end cap may shift, but the basic layout never changes. You can use this to your advantage. Make a list before you go. Be specific; instead of writing "snacks" and winding up with the entire Dolly Madison collection in your cart, write "yogurt" or "sliced almonds." This way, you'll be able to make tactical strikes; quickly buy exactly what you need instead of the crap they're trying to foist off on you. Here's your guide to sneaking past the schlock and marching down the aisle in style.

Produce: Work the Greens

Most produce is just as nutritious frozen as it is fresh, so be judicious. If you use it up slowly, pack your freezer. If you burn through greens like Vijay Singh, stick with fresh (taste and texture will be better).

Fresh strawberries and blueberries: Don't think you'll finish them in 3 to 5 days? Buy frozen instead.

Bananas: Avoid too-green ones. They'll add a strange tang to a smoothie.

Green onions: Green onions are much easier to use than whole onions for small meals. Just chop the tops and toss the bulb—no half-cut-up, plastic-wrapped onions stinking up your fridge.

Bagged baby spinach leaves: Peer through the bottom of the bag. If you see any mush, choose another one.

Broccoli: Look for tights buds or florets; they indicate a fresher find.

Cucumbers: Choose English cucumbers. They're longer and thinner than ordinary ones and usually come wrapped individually in plastic. Buy them for the convenience factor; they have hardly any seeds.

Peppers: Avoid peppers with wrinkled skin; it means they're starting to age.

Tomatoes: When possible, buy vine-ripened over hot-house. You don't have to be a gourmand to notice the improvement in taste and texture.

Lemons: Pick fruits that feel heavy; it means they have more juice.

Mixed-green salad blend: The more colors, the more antioxidants. Look for one with red radicchio, pale green endive, and dark-green spinach.

Avocados: The blacker, the better. Too green and they won't be ripe enough to eat.

Fresh cilantro: Tear off a leaf and taste it to make sure you're buying cilantro and not flat-leaf parsley. Unless you don't like cilantro. In that case, buy flat-leaf parsley and use it instead.

Nuts: Buy unroasted and unsalted loose nuts by the pound so you're not getting more sodium than you bargain for.

Meat: Your Muscle Maker

While turkey is a top-shelf Powerfood, that doesn't mean other meats are off-limits. The key is getting the leanest protein for the least amount of saturated fat. Turkey does the job exceptionally well, but only if you buy breast meat. Mixed ground turkey, usually made from dark meat, can contain as much saturated fat as beef.

Fresh salmon: Ask for wild-caught salmon; it has fewer chemicals.

Fresh turkey or chicken cutlets: Check the label for sodium; some raw meats are plumped with a sodium solution—added salt you don't need. Look for one that contains less than 10 percent broth solution.

Ground turkey: If it's not made from ground turkey breast, it could have as much fat as beef.

Precooked chicken strips: Try Perdue Short Cuts. No painted-on grill stripes or strange chicken-from-concentrate texture.

Deli slices: Healthy Choice turkey or ham have next-to-nothing fat. For a little less sodium, chose plain or honey-roasted over smoked flavors.

Smoked salmon: This is a high-sodium food, courtesy of the smoking. Pick the one with the lowest levels.

Canadian bacon: Buy the thin-sliced varieties; a smaller piece will help you keep the sodium tab down.

Flank steak: Pick the one with the bluest tinge. That means it's aged enough for extra flavor, but it's not too old.

Lean ground beef: You want 95 percent lean; it's the one with the least amount of saturated fat.

Pork loin cuts: Get the thin ones; they cook in half the time.

Dairy: The Great White Help

Dairy products play a key role in the Abs Diet—as snacks, drinks, and as important ingredients in smoothies. They're your greatest source of calcium—the mineral more and more studies point to as a key weight-loss ingredient—and pack a potent protein punch as well. Think of the dairy section as fat-loss central. If you play the percentages.

THE BEST PREPARED FOOD YOU CAN BUY. PERIOD.

Rotisserie chicken is an amazing thing. Not only does it look impressive, but it's an incredibly smart buy, both for the diet- and budget-conscious. First, always purchase a plain one; you're going to pick the skin off anyway, since that's where most of the fat hides. A breast and a leg will make a fine meal (check out the nutrition numbers below). Use the meat that's left to make a chicken salad or stuff it into a quesadilla. And then, toss the entire carcass into a stockpot full of water with chopped vegetables and spices of your choice, simmer for a couple of hours, and you'll wind up with the best chicken soup you've ever eaten. (Just fish out the bones before digging in.)

3 ounces breast meat (without skin)
120 calories, 1.5 g fat (0.5 g saturated), 65 mg sodium

3 ounces dark meat (without skin)
130 calories, 4 g fat (1 g saturated), 80 mg sodium

Low-fat milk: Horizon Organic. Cow antibiotics are for sick cows. Go organic.

Chocolate milk: Choose Horizon Organic Reduced-Fat in stow-and-go boxes. They don't require refrigeration, so you can take a healthy source of calcium and protein with you anywhere.

Eggs: Eggland's Best omega-3 fortified eggs provide an extra shot of heart-healthy omega-3 fatty acids.

Reduced-fat yogurt: Stonyfield Farm 100 Percent organic has just-right creamy texture.

Shredded cheeses: Sargento Reduced Fat shredded cheese blends offers the best taste for the least fat. Plus, they melt evenly, unlike most other reduced-fat cheese.

Part-skim ricotta cheese: Get the big tub. It doesn't expire quickly, and you'll finish it long before it threatens to go bad. Ricotta is a great natural source of whey protein, one of nature's premium muscle-builders.

String cheese: Sorrento Stringsters has 8 grams of muscle-building protein per stick, plus more calcium than other brands.

Cottage cheese: Cottage cheese is a stealth-sodium food; choose Friendship All-Natural Low-Fat No Salt Added and save the salt for something else.

Pudding cups: Swiss Miss. Ordinarily, you should watch out for added sugar. But no-sugar-added pudding is just nasty. This one only has 25 grams of sugary carbs, which won't kill you or blow the diet. As long as you just eat one. Occasionally.

Back-up smoothie: Stonyfield Farm has no high-fructose corn syrup, which can't be said for many other bottled smoothies.

Canned Foods: What's in Storage

Canned foods last will outlast your grandchildren, which is why they're used for currency in so many postapocalypse movies. Just watch out for sodium, the main preservative.

Tuna: Star Kist Premium Chunk White Albacore Tuna in

Water. Water cuts the fat. But the no-draining-needed bag seals the deal.

Salmon: Tulip brand has more fat than others, but it also tastes like salmon and not canned tuna.

Garbanzos, black beans, kidney beans: You can't go wrong. But before you cook with them, always rinse off the salty solution they soak in.

Chicken broth: Swanson Fat-Free Reduced Sodium tastes like the chicken, not like the can it came in.

Marinara: Muir Glen Italian Herb is preseasoned, so you don't have to spice it up. And it's not loaded with high-fructose corn syrup like other varieties.

Canned tomatoes: Del Monte Diced Tomatoes, No Salt Added is low sodium and, unlike other brands, contains no high-fructose corn syrup.

Peaches: Buy Dole sliced peaches, simply because they come in a resealable plastic jar. No fooling with a can opener or Tupperware.

Pumpkin: Buy the in-store brand. Since you're just going to dump it in a smoothie anyway, might as well save a few cents.

Sauces: Topping the List

Normally, sauces are like one-night stands. You enjoy them in the moment, but you feel pretty guilty afterwards. But I've uncovered some choice selections that might just make you interested in a lifelong commitment.

Olive oil: Choose extra virgin, which means the goods haven't been damaged by mixing with other oils.

Balsamic or red wine vinegar: There's no need to buy super-pricey vinegars shipped over from some forgotten enclave of the Mediterranean. Alessi is a quality, reasonably priced brand.

Soy sauce: At 560 milligrams of sodium per tablespoon, La Choy Lite keeps you from getting buried in a salt mine.

Hot sauce: Chohula is plenty potent, but it's not laced with extra sodium like many brands.

Peanut butter: Crazy Richard's Natural tastes exactly like roast peanuts. Not surprising, since peanuts—and a touch of salt—are its only ingredients.

Salsa: Walnut Acres Black Bean and Corn. Black beans provide a small protein boost, and corn contributes the antioxidant zeaxanthin.

Hummus: Asmar's Roasted Pepper. The peppers give you a little extra flavor to go with the 3 grams of protein.

Mustard: To me, deli-style mustards have more flavor than the sharp yellow kinds. Among them, Silver Springs Deli Style Horseradish has a nice extra kick, but barely any sodium (70 milligrams).

The Freezer: Cold Comfort

Shop here last and you'll likely make it home with your ice cream intact. "Ice cream?" you say. Right. This plan is designed for human beings rather than robots.

Fish: Gorton's Cajun Blackened Grilled Fillets are already spiced but not too salty.

THE LOW-FAT BUZZWORDS

Remember, food labeling isn't about education, it's about marketing. Labels can be confusing, misleading, and damaging if you don't know what you're getting into, especially when you're trying to figure out fat content. Here are some common phrases you'll see on food labels, and a look at what, exactly, they mean.

Regular: Greater than 3 grams of fat per serving

Reduced fat: 25 percent less fat than regular

Light or lite: One-third fewer calories or 50 percent less fat than regular

Low fat: No more than 3 grams of fat per serving

Nonfat or fat-free: Less than 0.5 gram of fat per serving

Shrimp: Since shrimp can be expensive, just pick the least expensive one. There's no real difference.

Waffles: Van's Gourmet Flax Waffles have slightly sweet whole-wheat flavor along with 1.6 grams of heart-healthy omega-3 fatty acids.

Berries and fruit: Choose Cascadian Farms organic. If you're buying frozen, it pays to go organic. Because they're delicate, berries and fruit often top the lists of high-pesticide produce.

Edamame: Make things easy for yourself and buy the already-shelled kind.

Ice cream: Edy's Grand Light is the hands-down best light ice cream on the market. It's sweet and creamy and has two-thirds less saturated fat than regular.

Condensed juice: Go with MinuteMaid. Off brands may have extra sweeteners.

Frozen Dinners

Frozen dinners can fit into nearly any diet for one reason: They're perfectly portion-controlled. (Well, except for the aptly named Hungry Man XXL, a size designation you're trying to avoid anyway.) In a study at the University of Illinois, people who regularly ate dinners from the freezer section lost 31 percent more weight than their free-eating counterparts. Plus, many of these meals include a respectable amount of fiber. And the 10 frozen dinners in this section in particular balance reasonable amounts of saturated fat with not-too-high sodium (a hidden danger of the freezer aisle).

LOOK! DOWN THERE! IT'S A BARGAIN!

More expensive items are typically found at eye level—right where you'll see them and sweep them into the cart without thinking. Look down, though, and you'll likely find a lower-priced version of the same thing.

Ethnic Gourmet:

Chicken Pad Thai

430 calories, 20 g protein, 71 g carbohydrate, 8 g fat (1.5 g saturated), 3 g fiber, 880 mg sodium

Healthy Choice:

Grilled Chicken Marinara

270 calories, 22 g protein, 35 g carbohydrate, 4.5 g fat (1.5 g saturated), 5 g fiber, 580 mg sodium

Grilled Turkey Breast

250 calories, 18 g protein, 31 g carbohydrate, 5 g fat (2 g saturated), 5 g fiber, 600 mg sodium

Grilled Steak in Roasted

Garlic Sauce

220 calories, 16 g protein, 22 g carbohydrate, 7 g fat (2.5 g saturated), 5 g fiber, 600 mg sodium

Lean Cuisine:

Chicken & Vegetables

240 calories, 19 g protein, 30 g carbohydrate, 5 g fat (2 g saturated), 2 g fiber, 630 mg sodium

Skillet Sensations Herb Chicken

250 calories, 15 g protein, 38 g carbohydrate, 4 g fat (1 g saturated), 4 g fiber, 890 mg sodium

Roasted Turkey Breast

270 calories, 12 g protein, 51 g carbohydrate, 2.5 g fat (.5 g saturated), 3 g fiber, 690 mg sodium

Smart Ones:

Beef Pot Roast

170 calories, 21 g protein, 10 g carbohydrate, 5 g fat (1.5 g saturated), 2 g fiber, 660 mg sodium

Stuffed Turkey Breast

270 calories, 13 g protein, 37 g carbohydrate, 7 g fat (2 g saturated), 5 g fiber, 720 mg sodium

Stouffer's:

Steak Teriyaki Skillet Sensations

190 calories, 11 g protein, 29 g carbohydrate, 3 g fat (1.5 g saturated), 4 g fiber, 950 mg sodium

Bakery/Grains: The Incredible Bulk

Fiber is crucial to weight loss, and the best place to find it is in whole-grain baked goods. If the first ingredient isn't "whole grain" or "whole wheat," keep looking.

LABELING LESSON

Any food label is like a store window. The front of it is designed to draw you in, and then once you're inside, you can figure out whether the product is worth it. With a food label, once you get past the pretty colors and the coquettish cartoon mermaid, you need to flip the can over and inspect the label. Here's what to look for.

Serving size: How much you consume. A common trick is for something that appears to be one serving (a bottled drink) to actually be two or more. Don't be fooled.

Calories: The measure of energy a food provides. Calories mean different things depending on what you eat, but in the end, extra calories that your body can't burn will get stored as fat.

Calories from fat: Multiply that number by 3. If that number is close to the total calories, it could mean trouble.

% Daily value: It's the percentage of the daily intake that the food supplies, based on a 2,000-calorie-a-day diet. A usually useless number.

Total fat: It's the combined total of saturated, polyunsaturated, monounsaturated, and trans fats. Look for a ratio that's at least 3 to 1, total to saturated. If monos and polys are listed, it's probably a healthy food. If it's more than 33 percent saturated or trans fat, consider another alternative.

Cholesterol: It's a fatlike substance from animals. Your body manufactures most of your cholesterol; what food adds is only a small percentage. Don't worry about it and don't get drawn in by otherwise unhealthy foods that claim "no cholesterol." As a nutritional selling point, it's worthless.

Whole-wheat bread: Pepperidge Farm or Milton's both offer a variety of high-fiber whole-wheat breads.

Tortillas: MexAmerican or Tumaro Honey Wheat are flexible enough for a wrap, yet sturdy enough for a quesadilla. Bonus fiber, too.

Pitas: Sahara Whole Wheat offers more fiber—5 grams— than other brands.

English muffins: Thomas' Whole-Wheat have a gram more fiber than the white-bread kinds.

Sodium: A mineral (salt, basically) added for flavor and to preserve foods. Unless you have high blood pressure or are sodium sensitive, use 2,000 milligrams as a reasonable daily target. More than that will not only raise your risk of hypertension, it will also make you retain water and look and feel heavier.

Total carbohydrate: This includes all of the sugar, starch, and fiber. Total number isn't as important as the kind.

Dietary fiber: The roughage that cleans your digestive and circulatory system. Insoluble fiber (in whole-grain foods, nuts, and beans) expands and takes up space in your belly, so it makes you feel full. Soluble fiber (in fruit and oats) keeps blood vessels lubed so cholesterol won't stick. Almost any food with at least 2 grams of fiber is good. Five is even better.

Protein: Amino acids that build and maintain your entire body. It helps you feel satisfied. Men who exercise should shoot for 162 to 225 grams per day—and women around 100. Thinner men need no more than 114 grams. Thinner women around 75.

Vitamin and mineral percentages: The food's percentage of the minimum amounts of nutrients required to prevent various deficiency diseases. As long as you're eating the ABS DIET POWER 12, you should be getting all the vitamins and minerals you need, but it never hurts to take a daily multivitamin for extra insurance.

Ingredients: Arranged in order by weight from most to least. Bad foods like high-fructose corn syrup and partially hydrogenated oils should be the fifth ingredient listed or lower. If not, move on.

Brown rice: Kraft Minute Rice Instant Whole-Grain Brown is ready in less than 10 minutes.

Pasta: De Cecco Whole Wheat is high in fiber, and this brand cooks well. It's not too tough or chewy.

Cereal: Here's your best chance for fiber. My favorites include: Nature's Path Optimum (10 grams) and Kellogg's Complete Wheat Bran Flakes (5 grams).

Oats: If your need is speed, choose Quick Quaker Oats. They cook in 1 minute and deliver 4 grams of fiber per half cup. If you have a little more time, buy Arrowhead Mills Steel Cut Oats. They take 7 to 9 minutes in the microwave, but they pack a potent 16 grams of fiber per half cup.

Baking: Piece of Cake

You'll have to navigate past the muffin mix and cake icing to find some important ingredients. Just grab your nuts and get outta there fast.

Nuts: Choose sliced almonds, chopped pecans, crushed walnuts—anything that'll slip into a bowl of oatmeal or smoothie and help save you time on the chopping block.

Honey: Buy the in-store brand. You'll use only small amounts, so there's no point in buying the super-expensive ones.

Spices: Here's another case where value rules. Despite what the label says, they'll last for ages, not just a couple of months. Get the cheap ones. You'll need basil, powdered ginger, cinnamon, cumin, and paprika.

Cookies and Candies: No-Sweat Sweets

Spend too much time here and you'll get fatter just thinking about all the sugar, HFCS, and lard that are lurking in these products. You'll have plenty of opportunity to satisfy sweet cravings—especially with smoothies that taste like shakes. But slip down this aisle for a few necessities.

Candy bars: Pick up York Peppermint Patties and Snickers in the bite-sized bags. The key part is bite-sized. Enjoying one or two after dinner is a pleasure no one should be deprived of, diet or not. You just have to supply the willpower to keep it at one or two.

Crackers: Triscuit Reduced Fat and Ryvita Crispbread are

FAT CONTENT OF MEAT (4 OUNCES, RAW, WITHOUT SKIN OR BONE)

	TOTAL (G)	SATURATED (G)
Skinless chicken breast	1.41	0.37
Veal steak	2.45	0.74
Wild rabbit	2.63	0.78
Lean ground beef	4	1.50
Cured ham	4.68	1.56
Wild duck breast	4.82	1.50
Chicken drumstick	5.05	1.34
Lean pork tenderloin	5.06	1.79
Beef sirloin steak	5.15	2
Beefalo	5.44	2.31
Turkey leg	7.62	2.34
Turkey breast	7.96	2.17
Lean beef tenderloin	8.02	3
Lean pork chop	8.19	2.85
Porterhouse steak	8.58	3
Lean ground turkey	9.37	2.55
Veal breast meat	9.73	3.80
Rib-eye steak	18.03	7.30
T-bone steak	19.63	7.69
Ham	21.40	7.42
Pork belly	60.11	21.92
Cured pork	91.29	33.32

the best whole-wheat crackers for fiber at 3 grams per serving.

Cookies: Fig bars—they're sweet and satisfying, thanks to the fiber. Fig Newtons have 1 gram of fiber per 2-cookie serving; Bakery Barbara's Whole-Wheat Fig Bars have 1 gram per cookie.

Drinks: Liquid assets

Loading up on soda or fruit juice is like reverse liposuction; it's pouring calories that'll be stored as fat back into your body. There's only one drink of choice, but you can spruce it up with a slice of lemon or lime.

Bottled water: Buy an entire case. That way, you can't ignore it. Take a bottle everywhere.

ABS DIET SUCCESS STORY

"IT DOESN'T EVEN FEEL LIKE A DIET"

Name: Jon Armond

Height: 6'4"

Age: 33

Weight, Week 1: 254

Weight, Week 6: 229

Weight, Week 9: 219

Body-Fat Percentage, Week 1: 27

Body-Fat Percentage, Week 9: 18

Jon Armond's a big guy, and he's always carried his weight well. When he told people he was trying to lose weight, they told him he didn't need to. But Armond knew better. Carrying more than 250 pounds around everywhere he went was taking a serious toll on his body, and he knew he needed to drop some serious pounds.

Even though he was active, Armond was one of those guys who rationalized that he could eat whatever he wanted because he had exercised.

Health food: Alternative routes

Most foods in the health food aisle or store taste like the box your computer came in—only worse. (Rice cakes? No thanks.) But there are some great finds lurking in the aisles, and you don't have to be a dietary masochist or an unreformed hippie to shop for them.

Flaxseed: Try Barleans's Forti-Flax. Buying your flax pre-ground saves time. And this one comes in a 16-ounce container that'll last for months. Look for it in the refrigerated section.

Whey protein: Look for protein powder that also includes casein, another dairy-based muscle builder.

But the fact was that he ate and drank too much, and he was always tired. (He frequently took naps in the middle of the day).

"I just didn't feel like I was 33," he says. "I felt like I was 53." Then he found the Abs Diet.

"When I looked in *Men's Health* and looked at the way the Abs Diet was set up, something clicked. This made perfect sense," he says. "I knew I'd lose weight, but what I didn't expect was the total-body transformation—to see the fat drop and the muscle gain at the same time. That's what I really appreciate about it."

For the first 6 weeks, Armond stuck to the principles without wavering, and he realized that it wasn't really a diet at all, but just a different approach to eating.

"I found myself not even consumed with it. I've never been on a diet that you didn't have to think about being on the diet all the time," he says. Instead, it was a plan that he simply incorporated into his life, and by doing so, he's traded in his "huge beer gut."

"I've got some abs showing through now," Armond says. "I was wearing size 38s, and I just bought 34s. I was wearing double-X shirts and now I'm wearing larges. I'm ready to go on the public-speaking circuit to talk about the Abs Diet."

Prepared Grocery-Store Foods

Remember when you were a kid, and all you had to do to score a heaping plateful of meat loaf and green beans was show up at the dinner table? The expanded deli sections of most upmarket grocery stores operate on the same principle. They cook it; you eat it. But this section of the grocery store is as littered with nutritional land mines as the rest (yeah, I mean you, crab cake). Here's how to chart a healthy path.

Heat-and-Eat Entrées

ABS DIET ENDORSEMENT:

Asian pan-seared salmon 250 calories, 12 g fat (1.5 g saturated), 350 mg sodium

THE LESSER OF TWO EVILS

Eat this: *Homestyle meat loaf* 230 calories, 11 g fat (4.5 g saturated), 470 mg sodium	**Not that:** *Crab cake* 500 calories, 32 g fat (5 g saturated), 990 mg sodium

ABS DIET SUCCESS STORY

A FORMER ATHLETE FINDS A BETTER BODY

Name: Mark Peterson
Age: 25
Height: 5'9"
Weight, Week 1: 187
Weight, Week 6: 170
Weight, Week 12: 164

Mark Peterson was a swimmer in high school and competed in triathlons. But then all that eating during college and law school hit him.

"Law school is the most unhealthy thing I've ever done in my life," he says. "I was looking for something to get me back in shape."

Heat-and-Eat Vegetables

ABS DIET ENDORSEMENT:

Asian-style bok choy 15 calories, 0 g fat, 190 mg sodium

Roasted asparagus and leeks 30 calories, 0 g fat, 130 mg sodium

THE LESSER OF TWO EVILS

Eat this: *Pesto vegetables* 70 calories, 3 g fat (0 g saturated), 190 mg sodium	**Not that:** *Creamed spinach* 90 calories, 4.5 g fat (2.5 g saturated), 460 mg sodium

Cold Sides

ABS DIET ENDORSEMENT:

Roasted corn salad 140 calories, 8 g fat (0.5 g saturated), 390 mg sodium

Bean salad 150 calories, 9 g fat (0 g saturated), 390 mg sodium

THE LESSER OF TWO EVILS

Eat this: *Orzo with vegetables* 180 calories, 10 g fat (0.5 g saturated), 570 mg sodium	**Not that:** *Tortellini salad* 300 calories, 26 g fat (1 g saturated), 660 mg sodium

He decided to train for the Chicago marathon and found a diet to support his training.

"The Abs Diet gave you a lot of different foods that you could have," he says. "It just seemed like a diet you could totally stick to."

He lived on almonds as a snack, spinach salad as lunch, peanut butter on whole-wheat toast before his workout, and made chicken or fish for dinner. "I didn't like oatmeal, so I substituted Kashi and Go Lean cereals."

In the fall, Peterson completed the marathon, and friends who hadn't seen him for months noticed the transformation. "They all said that it looked like I didn't need to lose weight and that I was crazy, but it's totally different when they see me now. A lot of friends couldn't believe the weight I lost."

Now that marathon training is over, he has another goal in mind. "I swam like crazy in high school, and I focused a lot on running, but I've never been close to a six-pack," he says. "This is the closest I've ever been."

Chapter 5

LET'S GET IT STARTED

25 Abs Diet Breakfasts

BEFORE WORK, there's a lot to do—take a shower, check the weather, dress the kids, glance at the stocks and scores, brush your teeth, zip the pants. In that routine, there's not much you can sacrifice—unless you want go to work in your skivvies. So many of us end up treating breakfast like it's a luxury—something that we do only if we have time or if there's a stale Pop-Tart on the floor mats. But sacrificing breakfast is like arguing with the cops; there's absolutely nothing good that can come out of it. Without breakfast, you're operating on reserves, putting your body in a pseudostarvation mode that tells your body's metabolism to slow down to protect you. What you need to do is eat—and eat heartily. Since I know you've apportioned about as much time to make breakfast as you have to slide on your socks, I've whipped up some recipes you can zip through faster than those artery-clogged lines at the drive-through.

So fire 'em up and start the day strong. What you eat the first hour you're awake will have a huge effect on what you eat for the next 16 or 17. I'm a firm believer that if every day of good eating is a race, then how well you start determines how well you finish.

Quicker Oats

USE PLAIN INSTANT OATMEAL for the following recipes. Nothing personal, Quaker guy, but those powdery sugared packets are as antiquated as that hat. For each recipe, mix all ingredients in a microwave-safe bowl and nuke for 2 minutes, unless otherwise noted. All serve 1.

Honey, I Shrunk My Gut (Powerfoods: 5)

1   cup 1% milk

¾   cup plain instant oatmeal

½   cup blue- or blackberries

1   tablespoon chopped walnuts or pecans

1   teaspoon honey

1   teaspoon ground flaxseed

     Dash of cinnamon

Per serving: 459 calories, 19 g protein, 70 g carbohydrates, 9 g fat (2 g saturated), 9 g fiber, 132 mg sodium

Flax Machine (Powerfoods: 4)

1   cup 1% milk

¾   cup plain instant oatmeal

½   banana, sliced

1   tablespoon peanut butter

1   teaspoon honey

1   teaspoon ground flaxseed

     Dash of brown sugar

Per serving: 515 calories, 22 g protein, 75 g carbohydrates, 13 g fat (3 g saturated), 9 g fiber, 172 mg sodium

You're Nuts (Powerfoods: 5)

1	cup 1% milk
¾	cup plain instant oatmeal
1	tablespoon chopped pecans
1	tablespoon chopped walnuts
1½	teaspoon honey
1	teaspoon ground flaxseed
⅛	teaspoon cinnamon

Per serving: 480 calories, 20 g protein, 63 g carbohydrates, 14 g fat (3 g saturated), 8 g fiber, 132 mg sodium

Ginger? Roger! (Powerfoods: 5)

1	cup 1% milk
¾	cup plain instant oatmeal
1	tablespoon sliced almonds
1	teaspoon honey
1	teaspoon ground flaxseed
½	teaspoon powdered ginger
1	tablespoon vanilla yogurt

Mix milk, oats, almonds, honey, flaxseed, and ginger in a microwave-safe bowl. Nuke for 2 minutes. Top with yogurt.

Per serving: 420 calories, 20 g protein, 62 g carbohydrates, 7 g fat (2 g saturated), 7 g fiber, 142 mg sodium

Instant Omelets

At a diner, an omelet is just code for "throw the leftovers in a pan with some eggs." At home, they're a quick source of protein—and a chance to boost your Powerfood count with one pan only. For all recipes, stir 2 eggs with a fork until white and yolk are well blended. Add the remaining ingredients. Nuke for 2 minutes and 30 seconds or until the eggs are firmly set. All serve 1.

Tom Tomelet (Powerfoods: 3)

2 eggs
1 slice turkey, diced
1 tablespoon shredded reduced-fat Mexican cheese blend

Per serving: 237 calories, 16 g protein, 3 g carbohydrates, 18 g fat (7 g saturated), 0 g fiber, 374 mg sodium

The Green and White (Powerfoods: 3)

2 eggs
1 tablespoon shredded part-skim mozzarella cheese
⅓ cup torn baby spinach leaves

Per serving: 221 calories, 15 g protein, 3 g carbohydrates, 16 g fat (6.5 g saturated), <1 g fiber, 256 mg sodium

Lean Eggs and Ham (Powerfoods: 2)

2 eggs
1 slice Canadian bacon, diced
1 slice tomato, chopped

Per serving: 271 calories, 23 g protein, 4 g carbohydrates, 18 g fat (7 g saturated), 0 g fiber, 781 mg sodium

Bean Counter (Powerfoods: 2)

2 eggs
2 tablespoons rinsed black beans
1 teaspoon cilantro

After cooking, top with 1 tablespoon salsa.

Per serving: 230 calories, 15 g protein, 8 g carbohydrates, 15 g fat (6 g saturated), 1 g fiber, 361 mg sodium

Up in Smoke (Powerfoods: 3)

2   eggs

1   ounce diced smoked salmon

⅓   cup torn baby spinach leaves

*Per serving: 236 calories, 18 g protein, 3 g carbohydrates, 16 g fat
(6 g saturated), 0 g fiber, 790 mg sodium*

The Mister Bean (Powerfoods: 4)

2   eggs

1   slice turkey, diced

1   tablespoon rinsed black or cannellini beans

1   tablespoon shredded part-skim mozzarella cheese

*Per serving: 240 calories, 17 g protein, 5 g carbohydrates, 17 g fat
(7 g saturated), <1 g fiber, 374 mg sodium*

Breakfast Burritos

You usually eat burritos for dinner, but a burrito is actually one of
the easiest things you can make for breakfast. Just arrange all the
ingredients on the tortilla, fold the ends, then neatly roll. For those
recipes that call for nuked eggs, you can scramble them in 60 seconds. In a microwave-safe bowl, just stir the eggs with a fork until
white and yolk are well blended and microwave for 1 minute per egg.

Holy Guacamole! (Powerfoods: 5)

1   medium whole-wheat tortilla

2   slices fat-free turkey deli slices

2   nuked eggs

½   avocado, sliced

2   tablespoon shredded reduced-fat Mexican-blend cheese

*Per serving: 494 calories, 25 g protein, 31 g carbohydrates, 35 g fat
(10 g saturated), 7 g fiber, 718 mg sodium*

Yosemite Salmon (Powerfoods: 6)

2 tablespoons part-skim ricotta cheese

1 medium whole-wheat tortilla

1 ounce smoked salmon, torn into little pieces

2 nuked eggs

1 cup chopped baby spinach

1 sliced green onion

Spread cheese on tortilla, then arrange remaining ingredients, fold ends in, and roll.

Per serving: 361 calories, 25 g protein, 26 g carbohydrates, 19 g fat (8 g saturated), 3 g fiber, 1026 mg sodium

Huevos Rancheros (Powerfoods: 4)

1 medium whole-wheat tortilla

2 nuked eggs

1 sliced green onion

1 tablespoon diced cilantro

2 tablespoons shredded reduced-fat Mexican-blend cheese

2 tablespoons salsa

Per serving: 326 calories, 20 g protein, 25 g carbohydrates, 19 g fat (7 g saturated), 2 g fiber, 713 mg sodium

DAIRY DAIRY, QUITE CONTRARY

At breakfast, put coffee in your milk instead of milk in your coffee. Fill your mug to the rim with fat-free milk first thing in the morning. Drink it down until all that's left is the amount you'd normally add to your coffee; then pour your java on top. You just took in 25 percent of the vitamin D you need every day and 30 percent of the calcium.

Breakfast Sandwiches

Once suitable only for the lunch box, today sandwiches might show up anywhere—as fancy canapés, as hearty dinner entrées, as sexual fantasies. . . . Okay, let's not go there. Right now we're concentrating on breakfast, so let's take a look at some healthy choices you can serve up in the A.M. (Who you serve them to is your business.)

Mex-illent Adventure (Powerfoods: 3)

1   tablespoons salsa

1   toasted whole-wheat English muffin

1   nuked egg

1   teaspoon diced cilantro

1   tablespoon shredded reduced-fat Mexican-blend cheese

ABS DIET SUCCESS STORY

HE LOST HIS POUNDS AND CURED HIS PAIN

Name: John Kelly

Age: 40

Height: 6'1"

Weight, Week 1: 215

Weight, Week 6: 193

When John Kelly was diagnosed with Barrett's disease—a condition caused by chronic acid reflux that can lead to esophageal cancer—he knew something had to change. He had a demanding job, three sons under the age of 9, and the stress of moving to a new house.

"It's hard to take care of yourself when there are so many other responsibilities that dominate your life," he says. Caught up in trying to be all things to all people, Kelly let his diet and exercise program slide, and, no surprise, he gained weight. "I just thought that gaining weight and being tired were par for the course."

Spread salsa on bottom half of muffin, top with egg, cilantro, and cheese. Toast in a toaster oven until cheese melts.

Per serving: 259 calories, 14 g protein, 29 g carbohydrates, 11 g fat (4 g saturated), 4 g fiber, 691 mg sodium

Foxy Lox (Powerfoods: 3)

- 2 tablespoons part-skim ricotta cheese
- 1 toasted whole-wheat English muffin
- 1 slice tomato
- 1 ounce smoked salmon

Spread cheese over each muffin half, top with tomato and salmon.

Per serving: 214 calories, 15 g protein, 29 g carbohydrates, 5 g fat (2 g saturated), 5 g fiber, 1027 mg sodium

But what wasn't par for the course were the unexplained pains in his chest. The pain was building to the point where he'd feel nauseous three times a week, and it got so bad that he had to skip work sometimes. When his doctor diagnosed Barrett's disease, Kelly began searching for ways to change his lifestyle, and he found some in the Abs Diet.

Because of the limitations he had with his illness—no fatty meats, spicy foods, or tomato sauce—Kelly found that the Abs Diet worked for him.

"My condition meant no vices—no alcohol or caffeine—so the idea of a diet that featured daily smoothies was pretty appealing," Kelly says.

Within weeks, the fat began to melt, and the muscles appeared. But it wasn't just the fat—or the fact that his energy levels had increased. Kelly wasn't feeling sick anymore—and hasn't experienced any symptoms since starting the diet.

"The Abs Diet helped me return to a more normal life on so many levels that the weight loss and fitness gain are just the icing on the cake," Kelly says. "Being able to contribute at my job and participate in my boys' lives more actively are blessings that I could have never imagined could come from a diet."

The Three-Country Breakfast (Powerfoods: 4)

1 nuked egg

1 slice Canadian bacon

1 slice tomato

1 toasted whole-wheat English muffin

1 tablespoon shredded reduced-fat Mexican cheese blend

Arrange egg, bacon, and tomato on one half of muffin. Top with cheese. Toast in a toaster oven until cheese melts.

Per serving: 326 calories, 24 g protein, 30 g carbohydrates, 13 g fat (5 g saturated), 5 g fiber, 1145 mg sodium

Apple Jacked (Powerfoods: 4)

1 toasted whole-wheat English muffin

1 slice Canadian bacon

2 slices apple

2 tablespoons peanut butter

Per serving: 403 calories, 23 g protein, 38 g carbohydrates, 20 g fat (3.5 g saturated), 7 g fiber, 1069 mg sodium

Jam Session (Powerfoods: 3)

1 toasted whole-wheat English muffin

2 tablespoons part-skim ricotta cheese

⅓ cup slightly crushed blue-, black-, or raspberries (mash berries in small bowl with fork)

Per serving: 197 calories, 10 g protein, 33 g carbohydrates, 4 g fat (2 g saturated), 4 g fiber, 460 mg sodium

Wafflewich (Powerfoods: 3)

1 whole-wheat toaster waffle

2 tablespoons peanut butter

¼ cup slightly crushed blue-, black-, or raspberries

Prepare waffle according to package directions. Spread peanut butter on waffle. Cup waffle in half, add berries, then squeeze lightly. Think of it as a berry breakfast taco.

Per serving: 308 calories, 12 g protein, 24 g carbohydrates, 20 g fat (3.5 g saturated), 5 g fiber, 212 mg sodium

Turk before Work (Powerfoods: 3)

1   whole-wheat toaster waffle
2   slices deli turkey
2   slices apple

Prepare waffle according to package directions. Arrange turkey and apple on waffle, then fold lightly in half.

Per serving: 139 calories, 7 g protein, 18 g carbohydrates, 5 g fat (1.5 g saturated), 2 g fiber, 359 mg sodium

Turbocharged Yogurt

In case you missed it (and I don't know how, since I've been jumping up and down and waving my arms about it for nearly 100 pages now), calcium is one of those ingredients that fortifies more than your skeleton. It seems to be a potent player in the weight-loss game. At breakfast, a cup of power-enhanced yogurt is the fastest power player since Mike Vick. For all, just mix the ingredients and eat.

Bananarama (Powerfoods: 2)

1   cup vanilla yogurt
1   banana, sliced
1   tablespoon chopped walnuts

Per serving: 363 calories, 15 g protein, 62 g carbohydrates, 8 g fat (3 g saturated), 4 g fiber, 163 mg sodium

Berry Easy (Powerfoods: 3)

1   cup plain yogurt

½   cup mixed berries

1   teaspoon ground flaxseed

Per serving: 204 calories, 14 g protein, 27 g carbohydrates, 5 g fat (2.5 g saturated), 4 g fiber, 173 mg sodium

The Rupert Pumpkin (Powerfoods: 2)

1   cup vanilla yogurt

¼   cup canned pumpkin

1   tablespoon chopped pecans

Per serving: 282 calories, 13 g protein, 40 g carbohydrates, 9 g fat (2.5 g saturated), 2.5 g fiber, 164 mg sodium

A Trip to the Peach (Powerfoods: 2)

1   cup vanilla yogurt

⅓   cup frozen or canned peaches (drain the syrup)

1   tablespoon sliced almonds

Per serving: 323 calories, 14 g protein, 55 g carbohydrates, 6 g fat (2 g saturated), 2 g fiber, 166 mg sodium

The Super Bowl of Breakfasts

Eight power foods in one bowl? We haven't seen this many A-listers since Oscar night. Start mixing.

The Ultimate Power Breakfast (Powerfoods: 8)

1   egg

1   cup 1% milk

¾   cup oatmeal

½   cup mixed berries

1   tablespoon chopped pecans or sliced almonds

1   teaspoon vanilla whey protein powder

1   teaspoon ground flaxseed

½   banana, sliced

1   tablespoon plain yogurt

In microwave-safe bowl, mix egg well, then add next 6 ingredients and nuke for 2 minutes. Remove, let cool for a minute or two. Top with sliced banana and yogurt.

Per serving: 587 calories, 30 g protein, 76 g carbohydrates, 15 g fat (5 g saturated), 13 g fiber, 254 mg sodium

Chapter 6

LEAN IN THE MIDDLE

25 Abs Diet Lunches

DEPENDING ON WHAT you do during the day, lunch can often present you with the opportunity to blow your diet like a tropical storm through the Florida Keys. Lunch comes at the very time of day when forces outside of our control are vying for our time. If your job is demanding, lunch sometimes means you have 3 minutes to pop the crackers out of the machine and get back to your desk. If you work with the get-some-fresh-air types, you're on the road at 12 and ordering a burger and beer by 12:06. If you need to have fancy business lunches, you're susceptible to the onslaught of free bread, creamy sauces, and four-story desserts. If you're home with the kids, you're one temper tantrum away from a macaroni-and-cheese binge.

That's why I suggest that if there's one meal that you should plan every day, it's lunch. Preparing for it makes you less likely to fall victim to any one of the diet busters waiting to pounce. It doesn't matter whether you make your lunch the night before, in the morning, or 3 minutes before you're going to eat it. The point is: Preparation breeds motivation.

Wraps

The trend toward sandwich wraps over the past few years has made eating a healthy lunch easier than ever before. An easy-access tortilla cuts down on empty calories and eliminates the need for utensils. But there are some bum wraps out there, so I've rolled up and rolled out a handful of smart choices just packed with Powerfoods. All make 1 serving.

Thai One On (Powerfoods: 4)

1½ tablespoons peanut butter

 1 whole-wheat tortilla

⅔ cup chopped precooked chicken

¾ cup mixed greens

¼ cup matchstick carrots

 1 teaspoon diced cilantro

Spread peanut butter down center of tortilla. Add chicken and remaining ingredients. Fold outside edges in, then roll.

Per serving: 331 calories, 29 g protein, 30 g carbohydrates, 15 g fat (2 g saturated), 5 g fiber, 661 mg sodium

The Day after Thanksgiving (Powerfoods: 4)

 2 tablespoons cranberry relish

 1 whole-wheat tortilla

 3 slices turkey

 1 slice Muenster cheese

¾ cup mixed greens

Spread cranberry relish down center of tortilla. Add turkey and remaining ingredients. Fold outside edges in, then roll.

Per serving: 311 calories, 24 g protein, 40 g carbohydrates, 11 g fat (6 g saturated), 3 g fiber, 1063 mg sodium

The Cow Tipper (Powerfoods: 3)

3 slices roast beef

1 whole-wheat tortilla

¾ cup mixed greens

¼ cup chopped tomato

1 tablespoon Dijon mustard

1 tablespoon blue cheese crumbles

Arrange beef slices down center of tortilla, then add remaining ingredients. Fold outside edges in, then roll.

Per serving: 208 calories, 22 g protein, 26 g carbohydrates, 5 g fat (2.5 g saturated), 3 g fiber, 1038 mg sodium

The Two Turks (Powerfoods: 6)

2 slices turkey

1 whole-wheat tortilla

2 slices cooked turkey bacon

¾ cup mixed greens

3 slices avocado

2 tablespoons shredded reduced-fat Mexican-blend cheese

Arrange turkey slices down center of tortilla, then add remaining ingredients. Fold outside edges in, then roll.

Per serving: 407 calories, 27 g protein, 32 g carbohydrates, 24 g fat (6 g saturated), 10 g fiber, 1376 mg sodium

Hot Curlers (Powerfoods: 4)

1 tablespoon Dijon mustard

1 whole-wheat tortilla

⅔ cup chopped precooked chicken

¾ mixed greens

¼ cup diced tomato

   Hot sauce to taste

2 tablespoons shredded reduced-fat Mexican-blend cheese

Spread mustard down center of tortilla. Add chicken and remaining ingredients. Fold outside edges in, then roll.

Per serving: 244 calories, 30 g protein, 28 g carbohydrates, 6 g fat (2 g saturated), 3 g fiber, 1089 mg sodium

Salads

Your standard chain-restaurant salad bar is a nutritional minefield—there are plenty of healthy, safe moves to make and plenty of fat bombs that can blow up your gut: potato salad, macaroni salad, croutons, those bacon bits that look like gravel. If you make your own salad, you can ensure that your salad has taste and power. All make 1 serving.

The Olympiad (Powerfoods: 4)

2½   cups mixed greens

  1   Roma tomato, chopped

  ¼   cup chopped cucumber

  1   tablespoon shredded part-skim mozzarella cheese

      Pinch black pepper

  1   tablespoon balsamic vinegar or red wine

  1   teaspoon olive oil

Per serving: 109 calories, 5 g protein, 8 g carbohydrates, 6 g fat (1.6 g saturated), 4 g fiber, 77 mg sodium

DIY DRESSINGS

Ever wondered how something that should by all laws of nature be refrigerated—like blue cheese dressing—manages to stay out on shelves? Trans fat and lots of preservatives do the work, making salad dressings some of the biggest belly-bloating foods out there.

Making your own salad dressing is just a little bit harder than boiling water, but it will ensure that you're eating 100 percent healthy (and it'll taste better, too). Add 1 part olive oil to 2 parts acid, such as lemon juice, orange juice, vinegar, or wine. Stir it together to blend or just pour each one on the salad.

Sweet Cheeses! (Powerfoods: 5)

2½   cups mixed greens
 ½   cup berries (any type or a mix)
 1   tablespoon chopped onion
 1   tablespoon blue cheese crumbles
 1   tablespoon chopped pecans or walnuts
 1   teaspoon ground flaxseed
 1   tablespoon balsamic vinegar
 1   teaspoon olive oil

Per serving: 235 calories, 6 g protein, 24 g carbohydrates, 15 g fat (2.7 g saturated), 7 g fiber, 160 mg sodium

Orient Express (Powerfoods: 6)

2½   cups mixed greens
 ½   cup diced precooked chicken
 1   green onion, sliced
 ¼   cup chopped green pepper
 1   tablespoon sliced almonds
 1   teaspoon diced cilantro
 1   tablespoon orange juice
 1   teaspoon olive oil

Per serving: 214 calories, 23 g protein, 10 g carbohydrates, 10 g fat (1 g saturated), 4 g fiber, 437 mg sodium

Kidney Punch (Powerfoods: 3)

2½   cups mixed greens
 ¼   cup drained canned kidney beans
 1   tablespoon chopped onion
 1   tablespoon blue cheese crumbles
     Pinch black pepper
 1   tablespoon red wine
 1   teaspoon olive oil

Per serving: 184 calories, 9 g protein, 20 g carbohydrates, 8 g fat (2 g saturated), 9 g fiber, 154 mg sodium

Potion of the Ocean (Powerfoods: 6)

2½	cups mixed greens
6	frozen shrimp, defrosted
1	green onion, sliced
¼	cup chopped cucumber
¼	cup chopped green pepper
1	tablespoon lemon juice
1	teaspoon olive oil

Per serving: 112 calories, 10 g protein, 8 g carbohydrates, 5 g fat (.78 g saturated), 4 g fiber, 112 mg sodium

El Tequila Ensalada (Powerfoods: 5)

2½	cups mixed greens
¼	cup drained black beans
1	Roma tomato, chopped
1	green onion, sliced
½	sliced avocado
1	teaspoon diced cilantro
1	tablespoon tequila or, for the less stout of heart, lime juice
1	teaspoon olive oil

Per serving: 325 calories, 8 g protein, 22 g carbohydrates, 21 g fat (3 g saturated), 13 g fiber, 250 mg sodium

WEEKLY GRIND

Several of these recipes call for lemon juice. If you have real lemons on hand, you can use the rind for zest. Zest adds flavor, and according to a University of Arizona study, a tablespoon of it each week can help cut the risk of developing skin cancer by 30 percent. Another handy tip: After using half a lemon for juice or zest, toss the rest down the drain and let it clean out your rank garbage disposal.

Sandwiches

As far as ease goes, nothing beats a sandwich. Bread, meat, eat. Still, as drive-throughs and the Hilton sisters prove, just because something's easy doesn't mean it's smart. There are plenty of sandwich fixings, from mile-high corned beef to do-nothing-for-you white bread, that simply don't stack up. Still, we love the sandwich. The trick is to incorporate as many Abs Diet Powerfoods into your concoctions as you can. That means some whole-wheat bread, some lean meat, and some leafy greens if you want. You want to build the ultimate power sandwich that's filling and more well rounded than Anna Nicole Smith (circa 2003). To shake things up, try making these substitutions without the extra layer of guilt.

SANDWICH	SUBSTITUTE THIS	FOR THAT	ABS DIET ADVANTAGE
Abs Diet BLT	Turkey bacon	Regular bacon	59 fewer calories
	Reduced-fat sour cream	Mayo	2 more grams protein
	Baby spinach	Iceberg lettuce	3 more grams fiber
	Whole-wheat bread	White bread	
Abs Diet meatball sub	Turkey meatballs	Beef meatballs	194 fewer calories
	Part-skim mozzarella	Full-fat mozzarella	4 grams less saturated fat
	Whole-wheat roll	White roll	3.5 grams more fiber
Abs Diet po boy	Defrosted frozen steamed shrimp	Deep-fried shrimp	379 fewer calories
	Reduced-fat sour cream	Rémoulade	3.5 grams less saturated fat
	Baby spinach	Iceberg lettuce	3.5 grams more fiber
	Whole-wheat roll	White roll	
Abs Diet gyro	Lean roast beef	Lamb	14 fewer calories
	Reduced-fat yogurt	Full-fat yogurt	1.5 grams less saturated fat
	Whole-wheat pita	White pita	3 grams more fiber

SANDWICH	SUBSTITUTE THIS	FOR THAT	ABS DIET ADVANTAGE
Abs Diet PB&J	Natural peanut butter	Trans-fatty kind	74 fewer calories
	Slightly crushed fresh berries	Sugary jelly	1 gram less saturated fat
	Whole-wheat bread	White bread	4 grams more fiber

Fill-in-the-Blank-Salad Sandwich (Powerfoods: 4)

6-ounces salmon or tuna or ⅔ cup chopped precooked chicken

1 green onion, sliced

¼ cup finely diced cucumber

1 tablespoon reduced fat sour cream

2 teaspoons Dijon mustard

1 teaspoon lemon juice

⅛ teaspoon lemon zest

Salt and pepper to taste

Mix everything together in a big bowl, stirring well to blend in the lemon juice and sour cream. Eat with mixed greens or whole-wheat crackers.

Salmon: Per serving: 149 calories, 19 g protein, 2 g carbohydrates, 7 g fat (2 g saturated), 0 g fiber, 661 mg sodium

Tuna: Per serving: 127 calories, 22 g protein, 2 g carbohydrates, 3 g fat (1 g saturated), 0 g fiber, 523 mg sodium

Chicken: Per serving: 118 calories, 20 g protein, 3 g carbohydrates, 3 g fat (.5 g saturated), 0 g fiber, 603 mg sodium

Soups

Soup is not the kind of food you think of as fitting into a busy lifestyle, it's hard to stash in your briefcase, tough to eat on the train, and generally frowned upon at business meetings. But soup does offer one big convenience. You can whip up a batch, store it in the fridge, then nuke it the next day (and the next, and the next) for a hearty, healthy, power-packed meal.

Macho Gazpacho (Powerfoods: 3)

3	large tomatoes
1	cup peeled chopped cucumber
½	cup reduced-fat plain yogurt
1	teaspoon balsamic vinegar
1	teaspoon olive oil
1	teaspoon lemon juice
¼	teaspoon salt

Seed the tomatoes (cut a crosshatch in the bottom, hold over the sink and squeeze—most of the seeds will come out of the bottom). Core and chop them into rough chunks and chuck them, along with everything else, into the blender. Puree until smooth. Serve cold.

Serves 2

Per serving: 118 calories, 6 g protein, 17 g carbohydrates, 4 g fat (1 g saturated), 4 g fiber, 349 mg sodium

The Beaning of Life (Powerfoods: 3)

1½	cans drained or no salt added black beans
½	cup reduced-fat, low-sodium chicken broth
1	chopped Roma tomato
1	sliced green onion
1	tablespoon lime juice
1	teaspoon hot sauce
1	teaspoon olive oil
1	tablespoon diced cilantro
½	teaspoon cumin
	Salt and pepper to taste
1	tablespoon shredded reduced-fat Mexican-blend cheese

Dump everything except cheese into the blender. Purée until smooth, scraping the sides if needed. Pour into bowls and microwave for 2 or 3 minutes, stirring occasionally. Top with a pinch of cheese.

Serves 4

Per serving: 365 calories, 24 g protein, 60 g carbohydrates, 5 g fat (1 g saturated), 22 g fiber, 475 mg sodium

Pita Pizzas

Contrary to popular belief, pizza *is* a health food. The tomato sauce provides vitamin C and the anticancer nutrient lycopene; the cheese gives you a hit of calcium and protein; and any vegetables you toss on top bring extra helpings of vitamins, minerals, and fiber.

Unfortunately, most commercial pizzas are corrupted by excess oil, fatty pepperoni, and horrific mutations like "cheese-filled crust." Talk about turning a good thing bad!

On page 159, I've ranked the national pizza chains from healthiest to unhealthiest. But when you want a quick hit of pie, try these home versions for the taste without suffocating your organs in pepperoni. For all of them, spread sauce evenly over pita, then top with remaining ingredients. Bake in an oven preheated to 475°F for 4 to 6 minutes. All serve 1.

The Whitey Ford (Powerfoods: 5)

   1   small whole-wheat pita

       White sauce (stir together ¼ cup part-skim ricotta cheese, 1 teaspoon olive oil, ¼ teaspoon dried basil or oregano)
   1   green onion, sliced
   1   tablespoon part-skim mozzarella cheese
   ¼   cup diced precooked chicken; 1 ounce smoked salmon, chopped; or three slices tomato

Chicken: Per serving: 254 calories, 18 g protein, 20 g carbohydrates, 12 g fat (4.5 g saturated), 2 g fiber, 393 mg sodium

Salmon: Per serving: 254 calories, 17 g protein, 19 g carbohydrates, 13 g fat (5 g saturated), 2 g fiber, 827 mg sodium

Tomato: Per serving: 231 calories, 12 g protein, 22 g carbohydrates, 11 g fat (4.5 g saturated), 3 g fiber, 263 mg sodium

The Red Auerbach (Powerfoods: 3)

1   small whole-wheat pita

¼   cup marinara sauce

1   green onion, sliced

2   tablespoons part-skim mozzarella cheese

3   frozen turkey meatballs; 2 turkey slices, chopped; or ¼ cup chopped green pepper

Meatball: Per serving: 292 calories, 24 g protein, 27 g carbohydrates, 10 g fat (3 g saturated), 3.5 g fiber, 557 mg sodium

Turkey: Per serving: 169 calories, 10 g protein, 21 g carbohydrates, 5 g fat (2 g saturated), 3 g fiber, 676 mg sodium

Pepper: Per serving: 156 calories, 7 g protein, 22 g carbohydrates, 5 g fat (2 g saturated), 4 g fiber, 451 mg sodium

The Pancho Villa (Powerfoods: 2)

1   small whole-wheat pita

¼   cup salsa, with a little of the liquid drained

1   teaspoon diced cilantro

2   tablespoons shredded reduced-fat Mexican-blend cheese

¼   cup diced precooked chicken; ¼ cup chopped green or red pepper; or ¼ cup chopped avocado

Chicken: Per serving: 166 calories, 14 g protein, 20 g carbohydrates, 5 g fat (2 g saturated), 3 g fiber, 664 mg sodium

Pepper: Per serving: 139 calories, 8 g protein, 21 g carbohydrates, 4 g fat (2 g saturated), 4 g fiber, 430 mg sodium

Avocado: Per serving: 193 calories, 8 g protein, 23 g carbohydrates, 10 g fat (3 g saturated), 5 g fiber, 434 mg sodium

Chapter 7

START YOUR NIGHT RIGHT

30 Abs Diet Dinners

TYPICAL SCENARIO: For the first 10 or 12 hours of your day, your life is somebody else's, whether you're working for a boss or catering to your kids. And just about the time you finally finish feeding everybody else's needs, your stomach starts sending you signals that it's tired of being ignored.

When you work hard all day—especially if you're too busy to eat right—it makes sense that you'd want to reward yourself with a big plate of Whatever the Hell You Want, maybe washed down with a Manhattan and a couple glasses of wine. And dinners should be a celebration of sorts—there's nothing wrong with rewarding yourself for forging through another demanding day and taking time to surround yourself with family, friends—and food.

But you can have your reward without sacrificing your health or your waistline. How well you eat at dinner is in great part determined by what you ate earlier in the day. If you fuel your body throughout the day with four smart, sensible meals and snacks, you'll find you aren't ravenously hungry the minute you walk in the door or craving the half-a-pig special at O'Bloaty's Tavern. You can, instead, enjoy a hearty—and healthy—meal, either at your favorite restaurant or at home with one of these simple recipes. Instead of using dinner as an opportunity to get drunk on fat and sweets, use it as an opportunity to pack in as many of the POWER 12 as you can.

Burgers

Burgers don't have to resemble deep-fried hockey pucks. Make yours with lean beef or turkey, grill or broil it just the way you want it, and enjoy a protein blast that will fire up your fat-burners and stimulate muscle growth. Most grocery stores now carry whole-wheat hamburger buns, so your classic "junk-food" dinner can morph into a perfect diet food—without sacrificing taste.

The Official Abs Diet Burger (Powerfoods: 5)

1	egg
1	pound lean ground beef
½	cup oats
⅓	cup diced onion
½	cup chopped spinach
2	tablespoons reduced-fat shredded Mexican-blend cheese
	Salt and pepper

In a large bowl, whisk egg. Add everything else, mixing it—your hands are the best tool—until well blended. Form into four patties. Place burgers in a grill pan or nonstick skillet that's heated over medium-high. Cook 6 minutes per side or to desired level of doneness.

Serves 4 (Wrap any extra burgers in plastic and freeze them for later.)

Per serving: 263 calories, 27 g protein, 8 g carbohydrates, 13 g fat (5 g saturated), 1 g fiber, 416 mg sodium

Alaskan Burger (Powerfoods: 4)

1   egg (use omega-3 eggs to up the good-fat count)

1   can salmon, drained

2   diced pieces of whole-wheat toast

1   tablespoon ground flaxseed

Salt and pepper

In a large bowl, break open egg and stir. Add everything else, mixing it with your hands until well blended. Form into four patties. Bake in oven that's preheated to 375°F for 20 minutes, turning once.

Serves 4

Per serving: 230 calories, 23 g protein, 12 g carbohydrates, 10 g fat (2 g saturated), 2 g fiber, 590 mg sodium

Ciao Down Burger (Powerfoods: 2)

1   egg

1   pound ground turkey breast

2   crushed cloves garlic

⅓   cup drained canned diced tomatoes

1   teaspoon dried basil

¼   teaspoon salt

In a large bowl, whisk egg. Add everything else, mixing it with your hands until well blended. Form into four patties. Place patties in a grill pan or nonstick skillet that's heated over medium-high. Cook 6 minutes per side or to desired level of doneness.

Serves 4

Per serving: 147 calories, 30 g protein, 2 g carbohydrates, 3 g fat (.5 g saturated), .5 g fiber, 235 mg sodium

Chicken and Turkey

Ask a culinary adventurer to describe the flavor of any exotic dish, from frog's legs to turtle soup to medallions of rattlesnake, and chances are you'll hear it "tastes like chicken."

That's not a lot of respect given to the humble chicken and its larger cousin, the turkey. But these two birds are powerful sources of lean protein and great go-to options whenever you're stuck for something to eat. Try these simple concoctions out for size, and the answer to the eternal question, "What does it taste like?" will always be, "Tastes like I want more."

Faux Fried Chicken (Powerfoods: 3)

1   cup of high-fiber bran flakes

1   egg

     Hot sauce

2   boneless, skinless chicken breasts

Put cereal in a zip-top bag, seal, and pound the hell out of it. In a large bowl, whisk egg and desired amount of hot sauce together. Dip chicken breasts in egg mixture, then roll in crushed cereal. Bake in an oven preheated to 350°F for 20 minutes.

Serves 2

Per serving: 211 calories, 31 g protein, 6 g carbohydrates, 6 g fat (2 g saturated), 1 g fiber, 243 mg sodium

The Dijon Lennon (Powerfoods: 3)

2   boneless, skinless turkey cutlets

1   teaspoon olive oil

⅓   cup reduced-fat low-sodium chicken broth

1   tablespoon Dijon mustard

2   sliced green onions

     Salt and pepper to taste

Pound turkey cutlets to an even thickness. Heat oil in nonstick skillet over medium heat. Brown each side of turkey cutlets, about 3 minutes each. Add broth, mustard, onions, salt, and pepper, stirring well. Reduce heat to low. Simmer for 10 to 12 minutes.

Serves 2

Per serving: 140 calories, 27 g protein, 2 g carbohydrates, 3 g fat (.4 g saturated), 0 g fiber, 364 mg sodium

Chicken a l'Orange (Powerfoods: 4)

1	teaspoon olive oil
2	boneless, skinless chicken breasts
1	tablespoon orange juice concentrate
2	tablespoons low-sodium soy sauce
¼	teaspoon powdered ginger
1	sliced green onion
1	tablespoon sliced almonds
1	teaspoon diced cilantro

Heat oil in a nonstick skillet over medium heat. Add chicken and sear for 3 minutes per side. Add orange juice concentrate, soy sauce, and ginger, stirring to mix. Reduce heat and simmer for 5 to 6 minutes. Before serving, top with green onion, almonds, and cilantro.

Serves 2

Per serving: 179 calories, 25 g protein, 7 g carbohydrates, 5 g fat (1 g saturated), <1 g fiber, 572 mg sodium

Precooked Chicken

Precooked chicken—low in saturated fat and high in protein—is ideal for busy people. You can eat it plain, chop it up and toss it onto a salad for a quick protein boost, or cook with it. Just beware, though—in order to preserve the cuts for your ease of use, these chicken pieces are saltier than fresh, uncooked chicken. So add as little extra sodium as possible to your meal.

Que Sera Quesadilla (Powerfoods: 4)

2   medium whole-wheat tortillas

½   cup reduced-fat grated Mexican-blend cheese, divided

½   cup diced precooked grilled chicken

1   heaping tablespoon diced fresh cilantro

1   sliced green onion

    Salsa

Place 1 tortilla in a nonstick pan that's preheated over medium-low heat, and top with ½ of the cheese and the chicken, cilantro, and onion. Add remaining cheese and top tortilla, pressing down to flatten. Cook 3 minutes, then flip and cook 3 minutes more. Serve with salsa.

Serves 1

Per serving: 425 calories, 42 g protein, 43 g carbohydrates, 15 g fat (7 g saturated), 4 g fiber, 800 mg sodium

Gonzo Chicken (Powerfoods: 8)

2   cups bagged mixed-green salad mix

1   cup baby spinach leaves

⅓   cup rinsed garbanzo beans

½   cup diced precooked chicken

1   tablespoon chopped pecans

1   sliced green onion

3   slices avocado

2   teaspoons olive oil

1½ tablespoons balsamic or red wine vinegar

    Salt and pepper to taste

Mix greens, beans, chicken, nuts, and onion together in a bowl. Top with avocado, oil, and vinegar.

Serves 1

Per serving: 420 calories, 30 g protein, 27 g carbohydrates, 23 g fat (2 g saturated), 9 g fiber, 799 mg sodium

It Takes Stew, Baby (Powerfoods: 5)

2	cups roughly torn baby spinach leaves
½	cup diced red pepper
1	crushed garlic clove
1	teaspoon olive oil
1	can (10.5 ounces) cannellini beans, drained and rinsed
1	cup cubed precooked chicken
½	cup fat-free reduced-sodium chicken broth
	Salt and pepper

In a nonstick skillet heated over medium-low heat, sauté spinach, peppers and garlic in oil 2 minutes, turning frequently. Add beans and chicken. Sauté 1 minute more. Add broth. Simmer for 10 minutes. Add salt and pepper to taste.

Serves 2

Per serving: 311 calories, 27 g protein, 43 g carbohydrates, 4 g fat (.5 g saturated), 11 g fiber, 420.5 mg sodium

Steak

Red meat pulsates with amino acids, the cinder blocks of your body's architecture. In fact, steak is the best natural source of creatine, an enzyme that helps stimulate muscle growth. So unleash your inner carnivore, and you'll unleash your abs as well.

Fruit of Your Loins (Powerfoods: 3)

2   beef tenderloin steaks
1   teaspoon olive oil
2   cloves garlic
¼   teaspoon pepper
½   cup raspberries or blackberries
⅓   cup red wine
    Salt

Place steaks in a skillet heated over medium-high heat. Cook 2 minutes per side. Remove from skillet. Add oil, sauté garlic for 30 seconds, then add pepper, berries, and wine. Return steaks to pan and cook 4 to 6 minutes more (or until desired level of doneness). Add salt to taste.

Serves 2

Per serving: 341 calories, 19 g protein, 5 g carbohydrates, 24 g fat (9 g saturated), 0 g fiber, 130 mg sodium

Sergeant Pepper (Powerfoods: 4)

6   ounces flank steak (about half of one)
½   green or red pepper, cut lengthwise into strips
⅓   cup cashew pieces
2   sliced green onions
3   tablespoons reduced-sodium soy sauce
    Hot sauce, to taste
1   teaspoon sugar

Cut meat diagonally and across the grain into thin strips (freezing it for 20 minutes first helps a lot). Place in large zip-top plastic bag with all other ingredients. Shake well to combine. Place into a skillet that's preheated over medium-high heat. Cook for 5 to 6 minutes or until meat reaches desired doneness, turning frequently.

Serves 2

Per serving: 363 calories, 29 g protein, 14 g carbohydrates, 22 g fat (7 g saturated), 1 g fiber, 873 mg sodium

Steak Fa-heat-as (Powerfoods: 4)

6   ounces flank steak (the other half of the one called for above)

1   small onion, cut into eighths

1   green or red pepper, cut lengthwise into strips

1   small jalapeño pepper, cut into rings

1   teaspoon olive oil

1   tablespoon diced cilantro

⅛   teaspoon cinnamon

¼   teaspoon cumin

Salt and pepper to taste

Cut meat diagonally and across the grain into thin strips. Place in large zip-top plastic bag with all other ingredients. Shake well to combine. Place into a skillet that's preheated over medium-high heat. Cook for 5 to 6 minutes, or until meat reaches desired doneness, turning frequently. Serve with four whole-wheat tortillas and salsa.

Serves 2

Per serving: 310 calories, 24 g protein, 46 g carbohydrates, 8 g fat (2.5 g saturated), 5 g fiber, 458 mg sodium

Mighty Muffins (Powerfoods: 3)

1   egg

1   pound lean ground beef

2   tablespoons balsamic vinegar

½   cup oats

¼   cup minced onion

Salt and pepper to taste

In a large bowl, whisk egg. Add everything else, mixing it with your hand until well blended. Divide mixture evenly into a 6-cup nonstick muffin pan. Preheat the oven to 375°F and bake for 25 minutes.

Serves 3 (Wrap extras in plastic and freeze them for later.)

Per serving: 349 calories, 35 g protein, 13 g carbohydrates, 16 g fat (6 g saturated), 1.5 g fiber, 329 mg sodium

Aztec Casserole (Powerfoods: 3)

6	ounces lean ground beef
⅓	cup diced onion
1	crushed clove garlic
¼	teaspoon cumin
1¾	cup cooked brown rice
¾	cup salsa
1	tablespoon diced cilantro
2	tablespoons reduced-fat shredded Mexican blend cheese

Brown beef in a large nonstick skillet preheated over medium heat (about 3 to 4 minutes.) Add onion and garlic and sauté 3 to 5 minutes or until soft. Drain fat. Add cumin, rice, salsa, and cilantro, stirring to mix well. Reduce heat to low and simmer for 6 to 8 minutes. Top each serving with a tablespoon of cheese.

Serves 2

Per serving: 397 calories, 25 g protein, 50 g carbohydrates, 11 g fat (4 g saturated), 5 g fiber, 537 mg sodium

One-Pot Dishes

Most of us don't mind the cooking so much as we mind the cleaning, which is where these recipes come in. Everything gets cooked in one pot, which leaves you more time for *nip/tuck* reruns.

Three Amigos Chili (Powerfoods: 5)

1	tablespoon olive oil
1	small onion, diced
1	pound ground turkey breast
1	can diced tomatoes with jalapeños
1	can (10.5 ounces) each garbanzos, black beans, and kidney beans, drained

1   can (14 ounces) low-sodium chicken broth

¼   teaspoon each salt and cumin

⅛   teaspoon cinnamon

     Hot sauce to taste

Heat oil on medium-low. Add onion and sauté until soft (about 3 to 5 minutes). Add turkey and brown (about 5 minutes.) Add tomatoes with juice, beans, broth, and spices. Stir and bring to a boil, then reduce heat and simmer 20 minutes.

Serves 6 (Freeze the leftovers and save $5 by taking them for lunch.)

Per serving: 293 calories, 31 g protein, 32 g carbohydrates, 5 g fat (0 g saturated), 11 g fiber, 788 mg sodium

Hot-Headed Chicken (Powerfoods: 5)

1   teaspoon olive oil

½   cup diced onion

⅓   cup diced red pepper

1   egg

1   tablespoon reduced-sodium soy sauce

     Hot sauce to taste

1¾ cup cooked brown rice

1½ cups diced precooked chicken

Heat oil in nonstick skillet over medium heat. Add onion and red pepper. Sauté for 3 to 5 minutes, until onion softens. Add egg, stirring frequently. Cook for 2 to 4 minutes more until egg scrambles. Add soy sauce, hot sauce, rice, and chicken. Stir and cook about 3 minutes more, until dish is well blended and evenly heated.

Serves 2

Per serving: 413 calories, 33 g protein, 49 g carbohydrates, 9 g fat (1.4 g saturated), 5 g fiber, 846 mg sodium

Pot Luck of the Irish (Powerfoods: 3)

2	small pork tenderloins
¼	teaspoon olive oil
½	cup diced onion
½	cup red pepper
1	cup packaged shredded cabbage
1	small chopped tomato
⅓	cup low-fat, reduced-sodium chicken broth
⅛	teaspoon paprika
	Salt and pepper to taste

In a nonstick skillet, brown pork 2 to 3 minutes per side over medium-high heat. Remove pork. Add oil, onion, and red pepper, sautéing for 3 to 5 minutes or until onion softens. Reduce heat to medium. Stir in cabbage, tomato, broth, and spices. Add chops to skillet. Cook 10 minutes more, stirring occasionally.

Serves 2

Per serving: 272 calories, 23 g protein, 10 g carbohydrates, 16 g fat (5 g saturated), 2 g fiber, 60 mg sodium

Seafood

To quote the culinarily confused sharks from *Finding Nemo*, fish are our friends. Besides delivering plenty of lean protein, most fish are packed with the omega-3 fatty acids that help control cholesterol and your appetite at the same time. To be as sleek and energetic as a dolphin, try these no-hassle recipes.

No-Scrimp Shrimp (Powerfoods: 3)

24	large frozen shrimp, peeled and deveined
½	cup chopped baby spinach leaves

1 teaspoon olive oil

1 crushed garlic clove

½ teaspoon dried basil

Hot sauce to taste

Mix all ingredients in a large microwave-safe bowl, tossing well to coat shrimp. Microwave 1 minute. Remove and toss again. Microwave 1¼ minutes more.

Serves 2

Per serving: 91 calories, 14 g protein, 1 g carbohydrates, 3 g fat (.5 g saturated), 0 g fiber, 165 mg sodium

The Aqua Man (Powerfoods: 3)

½ cup trimmed asparagus

½ cup matchstick carrots

1 teaspoon olive oil

Juice of 1 lemon

½ teaspoon lemon rind

1 crushed clove garlic

Salt and pepper to taste

2 tilapia fillets

In a small bowl, mix vegetables with oil, lemon juice, rind, garlic, and salt and pepper. Arrange fish in a small, shallow microwave-safe baking dish. Pour vegetable mixture over each fillet. Wrap dish tightly in plastic wrap, pricking a couple of times with a fork or toothpick. Microwave for 3 to 4 minutes or until fish flakes lightly with a fork.

Serves 2

Per serving: 136 calories, 22 g protein, 6 g carbohydrates, 3 g fat (1 g saturated), 1 g fiber, 220 mg sodium

Fish Tacos (Powerfoods: 3)

2   frozen grilled fish fillets, Cajun- or blackened-style

4   small corn tortillas

1   cup chopped baby spinach

4   tablespoons reduced-fat grated Mexican-blend cheese

Salsa

Microwave fish according to package instructions. Slice fillets into strips, then divide evenly among four tortillas. Top with spinach, 1 tablespoon of cheese, and salsa to taste.

Serves 2

Per serving: 270 calories, 25 g protein, 29 g carbohydrates, 7 g fat (2 g saturated), 4 g fiber, 674 mg sodium

Hot Pink (Powerfoods: 3)

2   3-ounce cuts of fresh salmon

1½   tablespoons reduced-sodium soy sauce

1   teaspoon olive oil

Hot sauce to taste

¼   teaspoon powdered ginger

1   sliced green onion

1   teaspoon chopped cilantro

On a foil-lined pan, place fish on top oven rack under preheated broiler. Broil 4 to 5 minutes or until fish flakes with a fork. Mix soy sauce, olive oil, hot sauce, ginger, onion, and cilantro in a small microwave-safe bowl. Microwave on high for 5 minutes, stirring once. Remove fish from oven. Transfer to plate, then pour half of the soy sauce mixture over each piece of fish.

Serves 2

Per serving: 203 calories, 20 g protein, 1 g carbohydrates, 13 g fat (2.5 g saturated), 0 g fiber, 460 mg sodium

The Perfect Storm (Powerfoods: 3)

2	tilapia fillets
2	tablespoons mustard
1	egg
½	cup finely chopped pecans
	Honey

Spread each fillet with about 1 tablespoon of mustard, then dip in beaten egg. Roll in chopped nuts. Bake in an oven preheated to 350°F for 10 to 12 minutes or until fish flakes. When done, drizzle each fillet lightly with honey.

Serves 2

Per serving: 371 calories, 30 g protein, 13 g carbohydrates, 25 g fat (3 g saturated), 3 g fiber, 513 mg sodium

Pasta

Legend has it that Martin Scorsese took Robert De Niro to Little Italy and directed him to eat pasta in order to balloon up for the second act of *Raging Bull*. But that doesn't mean you can't eat noodles and still look fighting trim. Whenever possible, opt for the whole-wheat versions; they'll give you gut-filling fiber and help take out a hit on your cholesterol. But with all pasta dishes, the key is to avoid fatty sauces and pile your plate high with Powerfoods.

The You-Can Noodle (Powerfoods: 3)

10 or 12 frozen turkey meatballs

2	cups diced tomatoes with sauce
½	teaspoon dried basil
1	crushed clove garlic
4	ounces whole-wheat spaghetti
2	tablespoons shredded part-skim mozzarella cheese

Defrost meatballs according to package directions. Toss with tomatoes, basil, and garlic. Microwave 2 minutes, stirring once. Toss with cooked pasta and top with cheese.

Serves 2

Per serving: 410 calories, 39 g protein, 39 g carbohydrates, 11 g fat (4 g saturated), 8 g fiber, 557 mg sodium

"Alfredo, I Know It Was You . . ." (Powerfoods: 6)

1   teaspoon olive oil
½   cup part-skim ricotta cheese
¼   cup 1% milk
1   packed cup canned salmon, drained
4   ounces whole-wheat spaghetti
2   tablespoons shredded part-skim mozzarella cheese
    Salt and pepper

In a sauté pan or skillet, heat oil and garlic over low-medium heat for 1 minute. Add ricotta and milk, stir, then add salmon and simmer 5 to 6 minutes. Thin with additional milk if needed. Pour over cooked pasta and top with cheese. Add salt and pepper to taste.

Serves 2

Per serving: 311 calories, 27 g protein, 20 g carbohydrates, 14 g fat (6 g saturated), 3 g fiber, 543 mg sodium

The Pesto Résistance (Powerfoods: 5)

1   tablespoon olive oil
½   cup walnut pieces
1   crushed clove garlic
2   cups torn baby spinach leaves
1   teaspoon dried basil
    Salt and pepper to taste
4   ounces whole-wheat spaghetti
2   tablespoons shredded part-skim
    mozzarella cheese

Heat oil in nonstick skillet over medium-low heat. Add nuts and toast 3 to 4 minutes, stirring frequently. Add garlic, spinach, basil, salt, and pepper. Cook 3 to 5 minutes more, turning frequently. Toss with cooked pasta and top with cheese.

Serves 2

Per serving: 335 calories, 9 g protein, 17 g carbohydrates, 28 g fat (4 g saturated), 5 g fiber, 160 mg sodium

Side Dishes

No matter what your main course, it's always smart to build your side dishes from the ABS DIET POWER 12—whether it's brown rice, spinach, salad, or beans. But you have many other options, as well.

The Breathalyzer (Powerfoods: 2)

- 1 teaspoon olive oil
- 1 crushed clove garlic
- 3 cups roughly torn baby spinach leaves

Heat olive oil in a skillet on medium-high. Add garlic and sauté 2 minutes. Add spinach, sautéing 3 to 5 minutes until all leaves are wilted, turning frequently with tongs.

Serves 2

Per serving: 37 calories, 1 g protein, 4 g carbohydrates, 2 g fat (0 g saturated), 2 g fiber, 136 mg sodium

The Green Party (Powerfoods: 2)

- 2 cups fresh green beans trimmed into inch-long pieces
- 1 heaping tablespoon sliced almonds
- ¼ teaspoon lemon rind
  - Salt to taste
  - Juice of ½ lemon

Arrange beans, almonds, rind, and salt (in that order) in steamer. Squeeze juice over the top. Steam to desired texture (3 to 5 minutes for firm beans). Add more salt to taste.

Serves 2

Per serving: 54 calories, 2 g protein, 8 g carbohydrates, 1.5 g fat (0 g saturated), 4 g fiber, 290 mg sodium

Nuclear Orange Spud Missiles (Powerfoods: 1)

- 2   medium sweet potatoes
- 2   tablespoons finely chopped pecans
- 2   tablespoons raisins
- 2   teaspoons whipped butter

Pierce potatoes with a fork. Microwave on high for 6 to 8 minutes, turning once. Cut them open and top each with 1 tablespoon pecans, 1 tablespoon raisins, and 1 teaspoon butter.

Serves 2

Per serving: 192 calories, 3 g protein, 32 g carbohydrates, 7 g fat (1 g saturated), 5 g fiber, 57 mg sodium

El El Bean (Powerfoods: 3)

- ½   cup canned black beans, drained and rinsed
- 1   cup canned corn kernels, drained and rinsed
- 1   sliced green onion
- 1   teaspoon diced cilantro
- 1   teaspoon olive oil
- ¼   teaspoon red pepper flakes
  Salt and pepper to taste

Mix ingredients together in a bowl.

Serves 2

Per serving: 150 calories, 5 g protein, 24 g carbohydrates, 4 g fat (0 g saturated), 6 g fiber, 550 mg sodium

Jerry's Rice (Powerfoods: 2)

1   packet quick-cooking brown rice

Reduced-fat, low-sodium chicken broth

1   cup broccoli florets, cut uniformly to thumb tip–sized pieces

Follow packaged rice directions, substituting chicken broth for the recommended amount of water and adding broccoli after broth has been brought to a boil.

Serves 4

Per serving: 136 calories, 4 g protein, 27 g carbohydrates, 1 g fat (0 g saturated), 2 g fiber, 80 mg sodium

Chapter 8

SHAKE THINGS UP

27 Abs Diet Smoothies and Snacks

WE LIKE TO DRINK—whether it's beer, Gatorade, or shots off the bartender's belly. But all drinks are not made alike—and some drinks can really sabotage your diet (or your relationship, in the case of the belly shots).

While some drinks, like presweetened iced teas, sports drinks, and Bud, are laden with empty calories, the right drinks can jump-start your metabolism and top off your tank with a healthy dose of Powerfoods. If you've got 3 minutes to spare, you can mix up a Powerfood smoothie. Dump the ingredients in a blender, push the button, and whip up a frenzy of belly-busting nutrition.

The best thing about smoothies is their versatility. You can down a smoothie at breakfast, use it as a meal replacement at lunch, make it your late-afternoon snack to take the edge off before dinner, or have it at night as your dessert. For all recipes, first blend together any liquid ingredients (milk, yogurt, juice, etc.) and protein powder; this will help break down the grainy powder and make sure it's evenly distributed. Next, add mushy ingredients, like precooked oatmeal and fruit, then add ice at the end. For a thicker shake, you can toss in more ice cubes; you'll add volume without the calories.

Check Your Blackberry (Powerfoods: 5)

¾   cup instant oatmeal nuked in water

⅓   cup blackberries

2   tablespoons low-fat plain yogurt

2   teaspoons vanilla whey protein powder

1   teaspoon ground flaxseed

3   ice cubes

Makes 2 8-ounce servings

Per serving: 149 calories, 8 g protein, 23 g carbohydrates, 1 g fat (0 g saturated), 3 g fiber, 17 mg sodium

Choco-nana (Powerfoods: 4)

1   cup 1% chocolate milk

1   banana

2   tablespoons low-fat vanilla yogurt

1   tablespoon chopped walnuts

2   teaspoons chocolate whey protein powder

6   ice cubes

Makes 2 8-ounce servings

Per serving: 185 calories, 9 g protein, 31 g carbohydrates, 4 g fat (1 g saturated), 2 g fiber, 106 mg sodium

The Orangeman (Powerfoods: 3)

1 cup 1% milk

½ cup frozen orange juice concentrate

2 tablespoons low-fat plain yogurt

1 banana

2 teaspoons whey protein powder

6 ice cubes

Makes 2 8-ounce servings

Per serving: 241 calories, 10 g protein, 48 g carbohydrates, 2 g fat (1 g saturated), 2 g fiber, 84 mg sodium

Tirami-Smooth (Powerfoods: 5)

¾ cup part-skim ricotta cheese

2 tablespoons low-fat plain yogurt

1 tablespoon slivered almonds

2 teaspoons chocolate whey protein powder

2 teaspoons ground flaxseed

½ teaspoon finely ground coffee

6 ice cubes

Makes 2 8-ounce servings

Per serving: 207 calories, 15 g protein, 15 g carbohydrates, 10 g fat (5 g saturated), 2 g fiber, 134 mg sodium

The Endless Summer (Powerfoods: 4)

¼ cup 1% milk

¾ cup ready-to-eat cubed seedless watermelon pieces

½ cup strawberries

½ cup low-fat plain yogurt

2 teaspoons vanilla whey protein powder

3 ice cubes

Makes 2 8-ounce servings

Per serving: 92 calories, 7 g protein, 13 g carbohydrates, 2 g fat (1 g saturated), 1 g fiber, 66 mg sodium

Punk'd Pie (Powerfoods: 5)

½ cup canned pumpkin

¾ cup instant oatmeal nuked in water

¼ cup chopped pecans

2 tablespoons low-fat vanilla yogurt

2 teaspoons vanilla whey protein powder

1 teaspoon ground flaxseed

3 ice cubes

Makes 2 8-ounce servings

Per serving: 270 calories, 9 g protein, 29 g carbohydrates, 11 g fat (1 g saturated), 6 g fiber, 19 mg sodium

Lime Dancing (Powerfoods: 3)

½ cup frozen lime juice concentrate

1 cup 1% milk

2 tablespoons low-fat vanilla yogurt

1 banana

2 teaspoons vanilla whey protein powder

3 ice cubes

Makes 2 8-ounce servings

Per serving: 274 calories, 8 g protein, 58 g carbohydrates, 2 g fat (1 g saturated), 2 g fiber, 88 mg sodium

Honey-Pecan Smoothie (Powerfoods: 5)

½   cup 1% milk

½   cup low-fat vanilla yogurt

¼   cup chopped pecans

2   teaspoons whey protein powder

PACK SNACKS

For snacks, you can eat leftovers, smoothies, or smaller portions of the ABS DIET POWER 12. Make sure each snack contains one or two Powerfoods, one of which must be protein. (Note: Dairy options count as protein, too.)

Protein options

2 teaspoons peanut butter

1 ounce almonds, pecans, walnuts, or peanuts

3 slices low-sodium deli cold cuts

½ cup shelled edamame

Dairy options

8 ounces low-fat yogurt

8 ounces 1% milk or chocolate milk

1½ slices low-fat cheese

1 stick string cheese

Low-fat, no-salt-added cottage cheese

Low-fat yogurt smoothie

Fruit or vegetable options

1 ounce raisins

Raw vegetables (celery, baby carrots, broccoli) in unlimited quantity

1½ cups berries

1   teaspoon honey

2   teaspoons ground flaxseed

6   ice cubes

Makes 2 8-ounce servings

Per serving: 224 calories, 11 g protein, 18 g carbohydrates, 13 g fat (2 g saturated), 2 g fiber, 78 mg sodium

4 ounces cantaloupe

1 large orange

Whole-grain options

1 or 2 slices whole-grain bread

1 bowl oatmeal or high-fiber cereal

3 whole-wheat crackers

3 cups fat-free popcorn

1 granola bar

Dessert options

As long as you're pairing them with Powerfoods (like a glass of milk), these indulgences will add a taste of decadence to a healthy snack.

1 chocolate pudding cup

3 mini York Peppermint Patties

3 bite-size Snickers

½ cup reduced-fat ice cream

Desk-drawer snacks

These complete snacks balance complex carbs and protein for a one-and-done fast snack.

* Clif Bar (5 g fiber, 10 g protein)

* Erin Baker's breakfast cookies (6 g fiber, 7 g protein)

* Nile Spice Dried bean soups (11 g fiber, 11 g protein)

Mango Tango (Powerfoods: 4)

½   cup ready-to-eat cubed mango

⅓   cup blueberries

½   banana

½   cup 1% milk

½   cup low-fat vanilla yogurt

2   teaspoons vanilla whey protein powder

3   ice cubes

Makes 2 8-ounce servings

Per serving: 158 calories, 8 g protein, 29 g carbohydrates, 2 g fat (1 g saturated), 2 g fiber, 80 mg sodium

Honey-Nut Cheery Oat (Powerfoods: 5)

¾   cup instant oatmeal nuked in water

¼   cup 1% milk

1   tablespoon peanut butter

2   teaspoons whey protein powder

1   teaspoon honey

1   teaspoon ground flaxseed

6   ice cubes

Makes 2 8-ounce servings

Per serving: 206 calories, 11 g protein, 26 g carbohydrates, 6 g fat (1 g saturated), 4 g fiber, 51 mg sodium

Blue Velvet (Powerfoods: 5)

½   cup 1% chocolate milk

½   cup low-fat vanilla yogurt

½   cup blueberries

2 teaspoons chocolate whey protein powder

2 teaspoons ground flaxseed

3 ice cubes

Makes 2 8-ounce servings

Per serving: 140 calories, 8 g protein, 22 g carbohydrates, 3 g fat (1 g saturated), 2 g fiber, 92 mg sodium

The Peachy Keen (Powerfoods: 4)

1 cup 1% milk

2 tablespoons low-fat vanilla yogurt

½ cup frozen peaches

½ cup strawberries

⅛ teaspoon powdered ginger

2 teaspoons whey protein powder

3 ice cubes

Makes 2 8-ounce servings

Per serving: 152 calories, 9 g protein, 27 g carbohydrates, 2 g fat (1 g saturated), 2 g fiber, 83 mg sodium

Cheesecake in a Cup (Powerfoods: 4)

¾ cup part-skim ricotta cheese

¼ cup 1% milk

½ cup blueberries

½ banana

2 teaspoons vanilla whey protein powder

6 ice cubes

Makes 2 8-ounce servings

Per serving: 200 calories, 15 g protein, 19 g carbohydrates, 8 g fat (5 g saturated), 2 g fiber, 139 mg sodium

Juicy Fruit Juice (Powerfoods: 4)

1	banana
½	cup strawberries
½	cup 1% milk
2	tablespoons low-fat vanilla yogurt
⅓	cup orange juice
2	teaspoons vanilla whey protein powder
3	ice cubes

Makes 2 8-ounce servings

Per serving: 137 calories, 6 g protein, 27 g carbohydrates, 1 g fat (.5 g saturated), 3 g fiber, 49 mg sodium

Chocolate Factory (Powerfoods: 5)

1	cup 1% chocolate milk
2	tablespoons low-fat plain yogurt
2	tablespoons peanut butter
2	teaspoons chocolate whey protein powder
2	teaspoons ground flaxseed
6	ice cubes

Makes 2 8-ounce servings

Per serving: 219 calories, 11 g protein, 20 g carbohydrates, 11 g fat (2 g saturated), 2 g fiber, 167 mg sodium

The Chocolate Latte (Powerfoods: 4)

½	cup 1% chocolate milk
½	cup low-fat plain yogurt
½	banana
1	tablespoon peanut butter

½ teaspoon finely ground coffee

2 teaspoons chocolate whey protein powder

6 ice cubes

Makes 2 8-ounce servings

Per serving: 171 calories, 10 g protein, 20 g carbohydrates, 6 g fat (2 g saturated), 2 g fiber, 116 mg sodium

---

Abs Diet Trail Mix (Powerfoods: 4)

A ready-made power snack is an effective one: It gives you something to reach for when you're hungry, and it gives you good ingredients without guilt. Make this trail mix on the weekend, then keep stashes on hand at work and at home.

1 cup whole almonds

1 cup pecan halves

⅓ cup plain oats

   Cooking spray

2 tablespoons honey

½ teaspoon cinnamon

1 cup orange-flavored dried cranberries (Craisins)

1 large packet dried apricots

Preheat oven to 350°F. Place nuts and oats in a bowl and spray evenly with cooking spray (about 3 shots). Drizzle with 1 tablespoon honey and add cinnamon, stirring to coat. Spread nuts evenly on a pan and toast for 15 minutes, stirring occasionally. Once they've cooled, stir in the second tablespoon of honey and mix in the dried fruit. Divide into ¼-cup servings and place each into a zip-top bag.

Makes 9 to 10 servings

Per serving: 170 calories, 3 g protein, 18 g carbohydrates, 9 g fat (0 g saturated), 3 g fiber, 0 mg sodium

The Cinnamon Girl (Powerfoods: 3)

¾   cup instant oatmeal nuked in water

2   tablespoons low-fat vanilla yogurt

1   teaspoon honey

1   teaspoon ground flaxseed

⅛   teaspoon cinnamon

6   ice cubes

Makes 2 8-ounce servings

Per serving: 142 calories, 5 g protein, 25 g carbohydrates, 1 g fat (0 g saturated), 3 g fiber, 11 mg sodium

Peach Vacation (Powerfoods: 3)

¾   cup 1% milk

¾   cup frozen or canned peaches (drain the syrup)

2   tablespoons low-fat plain yogurt

2   teaspoons vanilla whey protein powder

6   ice cubes

Makes 2 8-ounce servings

Per serving: 150 calories, 7 g protein, 29 g carbohydrates, 1.5 g fat (1 g saturated), 2 g fiber, 71 mg sodium

Mint Chocolate Morning (Powerfoods: 3)

¾   cup 1% chocolate milk

½   cup low-fat vanilla yogurt

2   teaspoons chocolate whey protein powder

1   frozen Peppermint Pattie

2   teaspoons ground flaxseed

3   ice cubes

Makes 2 8-ounce servings

Per serving: 168 calories, 9 g protein, 26 g carbohydrates, 3 g fat (1.5 g saturated), 1 g fiber, 116 mg sodium

The Hawaiian Five-O (Powerfoods: 4)

- ½   cup 1% milk
- 2   tablespoons low-fat plain yogurt
- ¼   cup frozen orange juice concentrate
- ½   banana
- ¼   cup strawberries
- ¼   cup cubed ripe mango
- 2   teaspoons vanilla whey protein powder
- 3   ice cubes

Makes 2 8-ounce servings

Per serving: 154 calories, 7 g protein, 31 g carbohydrates, 1 g fat (.5 g saturated), 2 g fiber, 50 mg sodium

The New Zealander (Powerfoods: 4)

- 1   cup 1% milk
- 2   tablespoons low-fat plain yogurt
- 1   medium peeled kiwifruit
- ½   cup strawberries
- 2   teaspoons vanilla whey protein powder
- 3   ice cubes

Makes 2 8-ounce servings

Per serving: 110 calories, 8 g protein, 16 g carbohydrates, 2 g fat (1 g saturated), 2 g fiber, 83 mg sodium

The Almond Hammer (Powerfoods: 5)

½   cup 1% milk

½   cup low-fat vanilla yogurt

¼   cup sliced almonds

2   teaspoons chocolate whey protein powder

1   teaspoon honey

1   teaspoon ground flaxseed

6   ice cubes

Makes 2 8-ounce servings

Per serving: 179 calories, 10 g protein, 18 g carbohydrates, 8 g fat (1.5 g saturated), 2 g fiber, 79 mg sodium

The Nutty Professor (Powerfoods: 5)

1   cup 1% chocolate milk

2   tablespoons low-fat vanilla yogurt

1   tablespoon frozen orange juice concentrate

½   banana

1   tablespoon sliced almonds

2   teaspoons chocolate whey protein powder

2   teaspoons ground flaxseed

6   ice cubes

Makes 2 8-ounce servings

Per serving: 181 calories, 9 g protein, 29 g carbohydrates, 4 g fat (1 g saturated), 2 g fiber, 107 mg sodium

The Neapolitan (Powerfoods: 5)

¾   cup 1% chocolate milk

½   cup low-fat vanilla yogurt

¾   cup sliced strawberries

1   teaspoon ground flaxseed

2   teaspoons vanilla whey protein powder

3   ice cubes

Makes 2 8-ounce servings

Per serving: 154 calories, 9 g protein, 25 g carbohydrates, 2 g fat (1 g saturated), 2 g fiber, 114 mg sodium

The Whey-Too-Good Smoothie (Powerfoods: 6)

¾   cup part-skim ricotta cheese

¾   cup 1% chocolate milk

¼   cup chopped pecans

½   banana

2   tablespoons low-fat vanilla yogurt

2   teaspoons ground flaxseed

2   teaspoons chocolate whey protein powder

6   ice cubes

Makes 2 8-ounce servings

Per serving: 340 calories, 16 g protein, 30 g carbohydrates, 18 g fat (5 g saturated), 3 g fiber, 184 mg sodium

Abs Diet Sundae Parfait (Powerfoods: 3)

Yep, it's still a diet. The ice cream gives you calcium and protein with only a modest amount of fat and refined sugar. Indulge and enjoy!

½   cup reduced-fat chocolate or vanilla ice cream

¼   cup berries of your choice, slightly crushed

1   tablespoon chopped nuts of your choice

Starting with the ice cream, layer the ingredients in a small bowl.

Makes 1 serving

Per serving: 162 calories, 4.5 g protein, 25 g carbohydrates, 5 g fat (2 g saturated), 1 g fiber, 56 mg sodium

Chapter 9

EATING OUT, EATING RIGHT

The Abs Diet Restaurant Survival Guide

Eating out in a restaurant can be exciting, tempting, arousing . . . dangerous. Here's this seductive menu in front of you—pictures and descriptions of creamy pasta, juicy burgers, cheese-drenched potato skins. They're looking at you. They're daring you. They're whispering in your ear with soft, slow, raspy voices: "Order meeeeeee."

So you—a person of dignity and restraint, a person with serious goals and a desire to change your body—now have to decide. Do you give in to temptation? You know what's right—what's good for you—but the temptations are crying out to you: the smells, the specials, the free bread, the "save any room for Chocolate Death?" sales pitches. Oh, just this once won't hurt. . . .

No, it won't. But you're going to find yourself in restaurants again and again, still facing the same choices, still being lured by the same temptations. What do you do? It's simple: Look for the Powerfoods. And pull out your copy of *The Abs Diet Eat Right Every Time Guide*.

See, you don't have to sacrifice flavor to eat healthy, and you don't have to deny yourself a night out on the town. You just have to know which menu options deliver the most nutrition with the least number of empty calories and bad-for-you ingredients. To help you through the decision-making process, I've compiled a tireless compendium of nearly every major chain restaurant in the country, with the best and the worst choices each of them has to offer.

Fast-Food Joints

You've probably already figured out that the grilled-chicken sandwich is the default option when you don't know what else to order. But even the greasiest of junk food Valhallas offers more healthy choices than you might suspect. And even if nothing on the menu qualifies as a health food, you can still cut down on empty calories and saturated fat by ordering smartly. The goal is to stick to the plan, not bore yourself off it. One fast-food burger now and then won't kill you. Just beware of special sauces, dips, and salad dressings. They're often loaded with calories and fat. Stick to ketchup, mustard, or barbecue sauce. And when given the choice, a second burger is usually better than the side of fries.

Arby's

ABS DIET ENDORSEMENTS:
Hot Ham & Swiss Melt 270 calories, 8 g fat (3.5 g saturated), 1140 mg sodium

Grilled Chicken Deluxe 380 calories, 12 g fat (2 g saturated), 920 mg sodium

Arby-Q sandwich 360 calories, 11 g fat (4.5 g saturated), 1210 mg sodium

THE LESSER OF TWO EVILS

Eat this: *Arby baked potato with sour cream* 320 calories, 12 g fat (7 g saturated), 45 mg sodium

Not that: *Medium fries* 380 calories, 16 g fat (2.5 g saturated), 690 mg sodium

Eat this: *Martha's Vineyard Salad with almonds and raspberry vinaigrette* 501 calories, 27 g fat (6 g saturated), 830 mg sodium

Not that: *Market Fresh Roast Beef & Swiss* 780 calories, 39 g fat (12 g saturated), 1740 mg sodium

Baja Fresh
ABS DIET ENDORSEMENTS:

2 Baja-Style Charbroiled Chicken Tacos 360 calories, 8 g fat (1 g saturated), 460 mg sodium

Shrimp Ensalada 180 calories, 4 g fat (1.5 g saturated), 1010 mg sodium

THE LESSER OF TWO EVILS

Eat this: *2 Baja-Style Wild Gulf Shrimp Tacos* 380 calories, 10 g fat (1 g saturated), 700 mg sodium

Not that: *Chicken Enchilada plate* 770 calories, 24 g fat (10 g saturated), 2270 mg sodium

Eat this: *Charbroiled Chicken Baja Ensalada with salsa* 325 calories, 7 g fat (2 g saturated), 1150 mg sodium

Not that: *Burrito Ultimo with Charbroiled Steak* 930 calories, 37 g fat (16 g saturated), 2010 mg sodium

Burger King/Breakfast
ABS DIET ENDORSEMENTS:

Croissan'wich with egg 270 calories, 2 g fat (1.5 g saturated), 175 mg sodium

THE LESSER OF TWO EVILS

Eat this: *Croissan'wich with sausage* 380 calories, 27 g fat (9 g saturated), 630 mg sodium

Not that: *Croissan'wich with sausage, egg, and cheese* 520 calories, 39 g fat (14 g saturated), 1090 mg sodium

Burger King/ Lunch & Dinner

ABS DIET ENDORSEMENTS:

Chicken Tenders (5 piece) 210 calories, 12 g fat (3.5 g saturated), 920 mg sodium (Add 35 calories for BBQ sauce or 90 for honey.)

THE LESSER OF TWO EVILS

Eat this: *Medium Onion Rings* 320 calories, 16 g fat (4 g saturated), 460 mg sodium	**Not that:** *Medium French Fries* 360 calories, 18 g fat (5 g saturated), 640 mg sodium
Eat this: *Chicken Whopper* 570 calories, 25 g fat (4.5 g saturated), 1410 mg sodium	**Not that:** *Whopper* 700 calories, 42 g fat (13 g saturated), 1020 mg sodium

Chick-fil-A

ABS DIET ENDORSEMENTS:

Chargrilled Chicken Sandwich 270 calories, 3.5 g fat (1 g saturated), 940 mg sodium

Fresh Fruit Cup 60 calories, 0 g fat (0 g saturated), 0 mg sodium

THE LESSER OF TWO EVILS

Eat this: *Carrot and Raisin Salad* 170 calories, 6 g fat (1 g saturated), 110 mg sodium	**Not that:** *Small waffle fries* 280 calories, 14 g fat (5 g saturated), 105 mg sodium
Eat this: *Chick-n-strips (4 count) (fried)* 290 calories, 13 g fat (2.5 g saturated), 730 mg sodium	**Not that:** *Chargrilled Chicken Club* 380 calories, 11 g fat (5 g saturated), 1240 mg sodium

Chipotle

ABS DIET ENDORSEMENT:

Burrito with black beans, vegetables, lettuce, and salsa 600 calories, 18 g fat (3.5 g saturated), 2378 mg sodium

THE LESSER OF TWO EVILS

Eat this: *Burrito with black beans, vegetables, lettuce, and guacamole* 770 calories, 33 g fat (6 g saturated), 2248 mg sodium	**Not that:** *Burrito with barbecue, rice, lettuce, salsa, cheese, sour cream* 1120 calories, 51 g fat (20 g saturated), 2920 mg sodium

Dairy Queen

ABS DIET ENDORSEMENTS:

Grilled Chicken Sandwich 340 calories, 16 g fat (2.5 g saturated), 1000 mg sodium

Chocolate Soft Serve ($\frac{1}{2}$ cup) 150 calories, 5 g fat (3.5 g saturated), 75 mg sodium

THE LESSER OF TWO EVILS

Eat this: *2 Hot Dogs* 480 calories, 28 g fat (10 g saturated), 1460 mg sodium	**Not that:** *Chicken Strip Basket with gravy* 1000 calories, 50 g fat (13 g saturated), 2510 mg sodium
Eat this: *Small Chocolate Sundae* 280 calories, 7 g fat (4.5 g saturated), 140 mg sodium	**Not that:** *Medium Chocolate Malt* 870 calories, 22 g fat (14 g saturated), 450 mg sodium

Hardee's

ABS DIET ENDORSEMENTS:

Country Ham Biscuit 440 calories, 26 g fat (6 g saturated), 1710 mg sodium

Slammer 240 calories, 12 g fat (5 g saturated), 300 mg sodium

Hot Ham 'n Cheese 287 calories, 13 g fat (6 g saturated), 1100 mg sodium

Mashed potatoes 90 calories, 2 g fat, 410 mg sodium

THE LESSER OF TWO EVILS

Eat this: *Frisco Breakfast Sandwich* 410 calories, 17 g fat (7 g saturated), 870 mg sodium	**Not that:** *Loaded Omelet Biscuit* 640 calories, 44 g fat (14 g saturated), 1510 mg sodium

THE LESSER OF TWO EVILS (CONT.)

Eat this: *Cole Slaw* 170 calories, 10 g fat (2 g saturated), 140 mg sodium	**Not that:** *Medium Crispy Curls* 410 calories, 20 g fat (5 g saturated), 1020 mg sodium
Eat this: *Regular Roast Beef Sandwich* 330 calories, 16 g fat (7 g saturated), 1220 mg sodium	**Not that:** *Half Pound Six Dollar Burger* 1060 calories, 72 g fat (30 g saturated), 1860 mg sodium

Jack in the Box/Breakfast

ABS DIET ENDORSEMENTS:

Breakfast Jack 305 calories, 14 g fat (4 g saturated), 715 mg sodium

THE LESSER OF TWO EVILS

Eat this: *Sourdough Breakfast Sandwich* 445 calories, 26 g fat (8 g saturated), 875 mg sodium	**Not that:** *Extreme Sausage Sandwich* 690 calories, 50 g fat (17 g saturated), 1265 mg sodium

Jack in the Box/Lunch & Dinner

ABS DIET ENDORSEMENTS:

Hamburger 310 calories, 14 g fat (5 g saturated), 590 mg sodium

Side salad with low-fat balsamic dressing 195 calories, 9.5 g fat (4.5 g saturated), 880 mg sodium

THE LESSER OF TWO EVILS

Eat this: *Egg Roll (1)* 175 calories, 6 g fat (2 g saturated), 470 mg sodium	**Not that:** *Stuffed Jalapeños (3 pieces)* 230 calories, 13 g fat (6 g saturated), 690 mg sodium
Eat this: *Chicken Fajita Pita* 315 calories, 9 g fat (4 g saturated), 1080 mg sodium	**Not that:** *Sourdough Jack* 715 calories, 51 g fat (18 g saturated), 1165 mg sodium

KFC

ABS DIET ENDORSEMENTS:

Original Recipe Chicken Breast (with skin and breading removed) 140 calories, 3 g fat (1 g saturated), 410 mg sodium

Mashed Potatoes with Gravy 110 calories, 4 g fat (1 g saturated), 260 mg sodium

THE LESSER OF TWO EVILS

Eat this: *BBQ Baked Beans* 230 calories, 1 g fat (1 g saturated), 720 mg sodium	**Not that:** *Potato Wedges* 240 calories, 12 g fat (3 g saturated), 830 mg sodium
Eat this: *Honey Barbecue Sandwich* 300 calories, 6 g fat (1.5 g saturated), 640 mg sodium	**Not that:** *Original Recipe Breast* 380 calories, 19 g fat (6 g saturated), 1150 mg sodium

Long John Silver's

ABS DIET ENDORSEMENTS:

Baked Cod with cocktail sauce 145 calories, 2.5 g fat (1 g saturated), 490 mg sodium

Corn Cobette 95 calories, 3 g fat (0.5 g saturated), 0 mg sodium

THE LESSER OF TWO EVILS

Eat this: *Chicken Plank (fried)* 140 calories, 8 g fat (2.5 g saturated), 400 mg sodium	**Not that:** *Ultimate Fish Sandwich* 500 calories, 25 g fat (8 g saturated), 1310 mg sodium
Eat this: *Pineapple Cream Pie* 290 calories, 13 g fat (7 g saturated), 210 mg sodium	**Not that:** *Chocolate Cream Pie* 310 calories, 22 g fat (14 g saturated), 170 mg sodium

McDonald's/Breakfast

ABS DIET ENDORSEMENT:

Egg McMuffin 290 calories, 11 g fat (4.5 g saturated), 850 mg sodium

THE LESSER OF TWO EVILS

Eat this: *Sausage Burrito* 300 calories, 16 g fat (6 g saturated), 760 mg sodium

Not that: *Sausage McMuffin with Egg* 450 calories, 26 g fat (10 g saturated), 930 mg sodium

McDonald's/Lunch & Dinner

ABS DIET ENDORSEMENTS:

Chicken McGrill 400 calories, 16 g fat (3 g saturated), 1010 mg sodium

Side Salad with Low-Fat Balsamic Vinaigrette 55 calories, 3 g fat (0 g saturated), 740 mg sodium

Fiesta salad with salsa 390 calories, 22 g fat (10 g saturated), 870 mg sodium

Fruit 'n Yogurt Parfait (with granola) 160 calories, 2 g fat (1 g saturated), 85 mg sodium

THE LESSER OF TWO EVILS

Eat this: *Quarter Pounder* 420 calories, 18 g fat (7 g saturated), 730 mg sodium

Not that: *Big Mac* 560 calories, 30 g fat (10 g saturated), 1010 mg sodium

Eat this: *Chicken Selects (3 piece) (Add 60 calories for buffalo sauce, 70 for honey mustard)* 380 calories, 20 g fat (3.5 g saturated), 930 mg sodium

Not that: *Crispy Chicken Bacon Ranch Salad with dressing* 620 calories, 31 g fat (8 g saturated), 1560 mg sodium

Eat this: *Apple Dippers with Low-Fat Caramel Dip* 100 calories, 1 g fat (0.5 g saturated), 35 mg sodium

Not that: *Baked Apple Pie* 250 calories, 11 g fat (3 g saturated), 150 mg sodium

Taco Bell

ABS DIET ENDORSEMENTS:

Chicken Burrito, Fiesta style 370 calories, 12 g fat (3.5 g saturated), 1090 mg sodium

2 Ranchero Chicken Soft Tacos 540 calories, 14 g fat (4 g saturated), 1710 mg sodium

THE LESSER OF TWO EVILS

Eat this: *Bean Burrito* 370 calories, 10 g fat (3.5 g saturated), 1200 mg sodium	**Not that:** *Fiesta Taco Salad (without shell)* 500 calories, 27 g fat (12 g saturated), 1520 mg sodium

Wendy's

ABS DIET ENDORSEMENTS:

Ultimate Chicken Grill sandwich 360 calories, 7 g fat (1.5 g saturated), 1100 mg sodium

Side Salad with Low-Fat Honey Mustard Dressing 145 calories, 3 g fat (0 g saturated), 360 mg sodium

Chili (small) 200 calories, 5 g fat (2 g saturated), 870 mg sodium

THE LESSER OF TWO EVILS

Eat this: *Baked potato with sour cream* 340 calories, 6 g fat (3.5 g saturated), 40 mg sodium	**Not that:** *Biggie fries* 440 calories, 19 g fat (3.5 g saturated), 380 mg sodium
Eat this: *Jr. Cheeseburger* 310 calories, 12 g fat (6 g saturated), 820 mg sodium	**Not that:** *Spicy Chicken Fillet sandwich* 510 calories, 19 g fat (3.5 g saturated), 1480 mg sodium

Sandwich Shops

Always start with building the right base: whole-wheat bread if they have it (rye is also a good choice because it has nearly as much fiber). Then make smart choices—low-fat cheese (go easy on it if all they have is full-fat cheese); no fatty, salty cured cold cuts like pepperoni or salami; and top it with tomatoes and all the greens that bun can hold. And don't always trust the salads; many are loaded with saturated fats hiding in fried noodles, butter-soaked croutons, and goopy dressings.

Atlanta Bread Company

ABS DIET ENDORSEMENTS:

Roast beef sandwich 450 calories, 5 g fat (n/a g saturated), 980 mg sodium

Turkey breast sandwich 420 calories, 4.5 g fat (n/a g saturated), 1450 mg sodium

Greek chicken salad 210 calories, 10 g fat (n/a g saturated), 690 mg sodium

Garden veggie soup (cup) 80 calories, 1 g fat (n/a g saturated), 820 mg sodium

Country bean soup (cup) 140 calories, 1.5 g fat (n/a g saturated), 1040 mg sodium

Fruit salad 140 calories, 1 g fat (n/a g saturated), 15 mg sodium

THE LESSER OF TWO EVILS

Eat this: *Chicken Caesar salad* 310 calories, 11 g fat (N/A g saturated), 580 mg sodium	**Not that:** *Turkey Club Panini* 780 calories, 32 g fat (N/A g saturated), 2000 mg sodium

Au Bon Pain

ABS DIET ENDORSEMENTS:

Grilled Salmon Salad Ficelle 280 calories, 7 g fat (2 g saturated), 490 mg sodium

Turkey Tenderloin Ficelle 310 calories, 9 g fat (1.5 g saturated), 860 mg sodium

Small Garden Salad 50 calories, 1 g fat (0 g saturated), 10 mg sodium

Blueberry yogurt with granola and fresh fruit (small) 310 calories, 6 g fat (2 g saturated), 130 mg sodium

Chargrilled Salmon Filet with Yellow Peppers salad 300 calories, 7 g fat (5 g saturated), 420 mg sodium

THE LESSER OF TWO EVILS

Eat this: *Dijon Albacore Tuna sandwich* 450 calories, 10 g fat (4.5 g saturated), 800 mg sodium	**Not that:** *Clam Chowder in a bread bowl* 880 calories, 19 g fat (7 g saturated), 2500 mg sodium

Blimpie

ABS DIET ENDORSEMENTS:

6-inch Turkey sub 344 calories, 5 g fat (0.5 g saturated), 1551 mg sodium

6-inch Grilled Chicken sub 373 calories, 9 g fat (2.5 g saturated), 836 mg sodium

THE LESSER OF TWO EVILS

Eat this: *Vegi-Max sub* 395 calories, 7 g fat (1.5 g saturated), 982 mg sodium	**Not that:** *Buffalo Chicken salad* 390 calories, 28 g fat (7 g saturated), 1300 mg sodium

Einstein Bros. Bagels

ABS DIET ENDORSEMENTS:

Harvest Chicken Salad on Challah 400 calories, 9 g fat (1 g saturated), 520 mg sodium

100% Albacore Tuna on Artisan Wheat 400 calories, 9 g fat (1 g saturated), 520 mg sodium

Tortilla soup (cup) 170 calories, 2 g fat (0 g saturated), 1150 mg sodium

Jamaican Jerk Entrée Salad 340 calories, 10 g fat (1 g saturated), 650 mg sodium

THE LESSER OF TWO EVILS

Eat this: *Calypso Chicken Salad Sandwich* 460 calories, 9 g fat (1 g saturated), 1100 mg sodium	**Not that:** *Club Mex on Challah Sandwich* 620 calories, 27 g fat (10 g saturated), 1660 mg sodium
Eat this: *Low-Fat Minestrone (cup)* 120 carlories, 3.5 g fat (0 g saturated), 940 mg sodium)	**Not that:** *Caribbean Crab Chowder (cup)* 220 calories, 14 g fat (12 g saturated), 790 mg sodium)

Panera Bread
ABS DIET ENDORSEMENTS:

Smoked Turkey on Artisan Bread 590 calories, 16 g fat (1.5 g saturated), 2320 mg sodium

Asian Sesame Chicken Salad 330 calories, 17 g fat (2 g saturated), 1170 mg sodium

Low-Fat Vegetarian Black Bean soup (cup) 160 calories, 1 g fat (0 g saturated), 820 mg sodium

THE LESSER OF TWO EVILS

Eat this: ½ *Chicken Caesar Salad/Low-Fat Vegetarian Autumn Tomato Bisque combo* 360 calories, 20 g fat (4 g saturated) 1675 mg sodium	**Not that:** *Pepperblue Steak Sandwich* 780 calories, 38 g fat (8 g saturated), 2070 mg sodium *Broccoli Cheddar soup (cup)* 230 calories, 16 g fat (9 g saturated), 1000 mg sodium

Schlotzsky's Deli
ABS DIET ENDORSEMENTS:

Dijon Chicken Sandwich (small) 329 calories, 4 g fat (N/A g saturated), 1456 mg sodium

Fresh Fruit salad (small) 86 calories, 1 g fat (N/A g saturated), 22 mg sodium

California Pasta salad (small) 58 calories, 3 g fat (N/A g saturated), 250 mg sodium

THE LESSER OF TWO EVILS

Eat this: *Albacore Tuna Sandwich (small)* 334 calories, 7 g fat (N/A g saturated), 1230 mg sodium	**Not that:** *The Original sandwich (small)* 525 calories, 24 g fat (N/A g saturated), 1781 mg sodium

Subway
ABS DIET ENDORSEMENTS:

6-inch roast beef sub 290 calories, 5 g fat (2 g saturated), 910 mg sodium

6-inch savory turkey sub 280 calories, 4.5 g fat (1.5 g saturated), 1010 mg sodium

THE LESSER OF TWO EVILS

Eat this: *6-inch roast beef sub with provolone* 340 calories, 9 g fat (4 g saturated), 1035 mg sodium	**Not that:** *Meatball marinara sub with provolone* 550 calories, 26 g fat (13 g saturated), 1305 mg sodium
Eat this: *6-inch savory turkey with provolone* 330 calories, 8.5 g fat (3.5 g saturated), 1135 mg sodium	**Not that:** *Atkins-Friendly Chicken Bacon Ranch Wrap* 440 calories, 26 g fat (9 g saturated), 1550 mg sodium
Eat this: *Oatmeal raisin cookie* 200 calories, 8 g fat (2.5 g saturated), 170 mg sodium	**Not that:** *Peanut butter cookie* 220 calories, 12 g fat (4 g saturated), 200 mg sodium

Zabar's and other NYC-style delis
ABS DIET ENDORSEMENT:

Turkey or ham on rye with lettuce, tomato, provolone, and mustard 370 calories, 12 g fat (6 g saturated), 1900 mg sodium

THE LESSER OF TWO EVILS

Eat this: *Corned beef on rye with slaw and mustard* 380 calories, 20 g fat (5 g saturated), 1500 mg sodium	**Not that:** *Egg salad on white with lettuce and tomato* 750 calories, 60 g fat (11 g saturated), 900 mg sodium

Breakfast Places

I can't emphasize enough the importance of eating the moment you wake up. They call it "breakfast" for a reason—you've been fasting for the past 8 to 10 hours, and your body needs fuel. Eating immediately jump-starts your metabolism and starts you on your daily quest to turn fat into muscle. On the other hand, if you skip breakfast, even for a few hours, you signal your body to begin breaking down muscle for fuel. That's right: Every minute you wait between waking and eating is a minute more of muscle loss.

That said, sometimes the fastest way to add fuel to the fire is to swing by one of these joints (especially on those mornings where you wake up somewhere . . . unusual). As a rule, make sure they don't put full-fat milk in your coffee concoction, go with reduced-fat vegetable spread on your bagel, and never buy a pastry that's bigger than your head. In fact, if there's one food category I would ban if I could, it's pastries and doughnuts—or, as they're known by their technical, scientific names, "empty sugar calories fried in lard."

Breakfast Diner (such as Bob Evans, Denny's, IHOP, Perkins, or Shoney's)
ABS DIET ENDORSEMENTS:
2 poached eggs 148 calories, 10 g fat (3 g saturated), 294 mg sodium

Plain whole-wheat toast (per slice) 128 calories, 2.5 g fat (.5 g saturated), 160 mg sodium

Canadian bacon 44 calories, 2 g fat (.5 g saturated), 364 mg sodium

THE LESSER OF TWO EVILS

Eat this: *2 scrambled eggs* 170 calories, 11 g fat (3 g saturated), 482 mg sodium	**Not that:** *Western omelet with eggs* 520 calories, 39 g fat (13 g saturated), 1280 mg sodium

Eat this: *Plain English muffin* 139 calories, 1 g fat (0 g saturated), 229 mg sodium	**Not that:** *Plain biscuit* 280 calories, 12 g fat (3 g saturated), 760 mg sodium
Eat this: *Bacon (2 slices)* 72 calories, 4 g fat (2 g saturated), 54 mg sodium	**Not that:** *Sausage (2 links)* 250 calories, 22 g fat (6 g saturated), 370 mg sodium

Coffee Shop (such as Caribou Coffee, Dunkin' Donuts, Peet's Coffee, or Starbucks)

ABS DIET ENDORSEMENT:

Cappuccino with fat-free milk (12 ounces) 80 calories, 0 g fat (0 g saturated), 105 mg sodium

THE LESSER OF TWO EVILS

Eat this: *Latte with fat-free milk* (12 ounces) 120 calories, 0 g fat (0 g saturated), 170 mg sodium	**Not that:** *Latte with whole milk* (12 ounces) 200 calories, 11 g fat (7 g saturated), 160 mg sodium

NUTRITIONAL DETECTIVE WORK

Food labels are all well and good when you're cooking for yourself, but what about those occasional nights (okay, endless stream of nights) when dinner is dished up by some pimply-faced kid with a paper hat and a bored expression? How do you know what, exactly, is in that paper-and-Styrofoam-wrapped monstrosity you're eating? In the land of "special sauces" and "secret recipes," sussing out the nutritional realities of your favorite entrees can take a little detective work.

If the greasy floor beneath your feet is that of a national fast-food joint, the answers may be pretty easy to come by. Most fast-food restaurants post complete nutritional information on their Web sites. Many will also have posters hanging in some dim corner of the restaurant, if you're willing to search. Be aware of two caveats: First, these menus change all the time, so you need to make sure what you're ordering is what they've posted. Second, watch out for serving size and extra ingredients: At some chains, the numbers for the "healthy" salad don't include the fried Chinese noodles that come on top. Others give you the calorie count

Bagel Shops

Bruegger's Bagels

ABS DIET ENDORSEMENTS:

Honey Grain bagel 330 calories, 3 g fat (0 g saturated), 500 mg sodium

. . . *with Light garden veggie cream cheese* 60 calories, 4 g fat (2.5 g saturated), 75 mg sodium

THE LESSER OF TWO EVILS

Eat this: *Pumpernickel bagel* 320 calories, 3 g fat (0 g saturated), 600 mg sodium	**Not that:** *Salt bagel* 300 calories, 2 g fat (0 g saturated), 1540 mg sodium

for a serving of their dressing, but the package that comes with the salad can be two or even three servings, not one.

Chain restaurants that feature actual menus and waiters are a mixed bag. Some deserve applause: Panera Bread Company and Don Pablo's Mexican Kitchen provide complete nutritional information on their Web sites. Others deserve a round of jeers: T.G.I. Friday's for example, refused to give us a nutritional breakdown of some of their foods, even when I called their corporate headquarters and harassed them. Applebee's will tell you the calorie count of their Weight Watchers items but not their regular fare. What's up with that?

So check your favorite chain's Web site. Even if they only list total calories, that's enough to make an informed decision—when you read that half of an onion-blossom appetizer has 1600 calories, you can pretty much figure the meal should only be administered under a cardiologist's care. If you can't find the information you want on the Web, call their customer service line. They might be able to e-mail or fax it to you. And if that's not an option, well, tell them you want it to be.

THE LESSER OF TWO EVILS (CONT.)

Eat this: . . . *with Light plain cream cheese* 70 calories, 4.5 g fat (2 g saturated), 90 mg sodium	**Not that:** . . . *with Bacon scallion cream cheese* 100 calories, 8 g fat (5 g saturated), 105 mg sodium

Manhattan Bagel Co.
ABS DIET ENDORSEMENTS:

Spinach bagel 270 calories, <1 g fat (0 g saturated), 580 mg sodium

. . . *with Light vegetable cream cheese* 50 calories, 5 g fat (2.5 g saturated), 100 mg sodium

THE LESSER OF TWO EVILS

Eat this: *Rye bagel* 260 calories, 1 g fat (0 g saturated), 560 mg sodium	**Not that:** *Chocolate chip bagel* 290 calories, 2.5 g fat (1.5 g saturated), 530 mg sodium
Eat this: . . . *with Light raisin walnut cream cheese* 80 calories, 5 g fat (3 g saturated), 75 mg sodium	**Not that:** . . . *with French vanilla cream cheese* 100 calories, 7 g fat (4.5 g saturated), 85 mg sodium

Bakery (such as Au Bon Pain, Atlanta Bread Company, Bruegger's Bagels, Caribou Coffee, Einstein Bros. Bagels, Panera, or Starbucks)

ABS DIET ENDORSEMENT:

Biscotti 110 calories, 5 g fat (1.5 g saturated), 75 mg sodium

THE LESSER OF TWO EVILS

Eat this: *Fruit or Raisin Scone* 410 calories, 14 g fat (8 g saturated), 350 mg sodium	**Not that:** *Coffee cake* 570 calories, 28 g fat (10 g saturated), 310 mg sodium

Doughnut Shop

Dunkin' Donuts

ABS DIET ENDORSEMENT:

Plain glazed donut 180 calories, 8 g fat (1.5 g saturated), 250 mg sodium

THE LESSER OF TWO EVILS

Eat this: *Jelly-filled donut* 210 calories, 8 g fat (1.5 g saturated), 280 mg sodium	**Not that:** *Old Fashioned cake donut* 300 calories, 19 g fat (5 g saturated), 330 mg sodium

Krispy Kreme

ABS DIET ENDORSEMENT:

Original glazed donut 200 calories, 12 g fat (3 g saturated), 95 mg sodium

THE LESSER OF TWO EVILS

Eat this: *Maple iced glazed donut* 240 calories, 12 g fat (3 g saturated), 100 mg sodium	**Not that:** *Dulce de leche* 290 calories, 18 g fat (4.5 g saturated), 160 mg sodium

Sit-Down Restaurants

Here's the big secret about those casual-dinner chain restaurants: They're really all the same place. Sure, there are some slight variations—Ruby Tuesday may give its spinach dip the pedestrian name while T.G.I. Friday's dubs theirs "Tuscan"—but both are the same vat of once-healthy vegetables sunk in saturated fat. The same principle applies to steak houses—a sirloin is a sirloin is a sirloin; maybe one place offers it in a 10-ounce cut while another in 12 ounces, but the meat remains the same. So even though these recommendations are not keyed to a specific restaurant, you can use them anywhere. At the steak house, look for cuts with "loin" in its name.

Steak House

ABS DIET ENDORSEMENTS:

Filet, aka tenderloin (9 ounces) 360 calories, 19 g fat (10 g saturated), 330 mg sodium

Barbecued chicken breast (10 ounces) 280 calories, 5 g fat (2 g saturated), 860 mg sodium

Steamed mixed vegetables 70 calories, 1 g fat (0 g saturated), 900 mg sodium

Side salad with light dressing 200 calories, 9 g fat (1 g saturated), 51 mg sodium

THE LESSER OF TWO EVILS

Eat this: *Sirloin (12 ounces)* 410 calories, 18 g fat (9 g saturated), 470 mg sodium	**Not that:** *Prime rib (16 ounces)* 1280 calories, 94 g fat (52 g saturated), 620 mg sodium
Eat this: *Sautéed mushrooms* 115 calories, 9 g fat (2 g saturated), 600 mg sodium	**Not that:** *Steak fries* 590 calories, 31 g fat (12 g saturated), 460 mg sodium
Eat this: *Baked potato with sour cream* 280 calories, 3 g fat (2 g saturated), 200 mg sodium	**Not that:** *Side Caesar salad* 310 calories, 26 g fat (7 g saturated), 620 mg sodium

Casual Sit-Down (such as Applebee's, Bennigan's, Cheesecake Factory, Friendly's, Perkins, O'Charley's, Ruby Tuesday, T.G.I. Friday's, or pretty much any restaurant with an apostrophe s)

ABS DIET ENDORSEMENTS:

Vegetable Soup (cup) 100 calories, 1 g fat (0 g saturated), 610 mg sodium

Grilled chicken (6 ounces) 270 calories, 8 g fat (3 g saturated), 650 mg sodium

Grilled salmon (8 ounces) 420 calories, 21 g fat (4 g saturated), 340 mg sodium

Vegetable of the day 60 calories, 3 g fat (1 g saturated), 150 mg sodium

THE LESSER OF TWO EVILS

Eat this: *Steak fajitas with salsa* 860 calories, 31 g fat (12 g saturated), 1660 mg sodium	**Not that:** *Rack of ribs (16 ounces)* 770 calories, 54 g fat (21 g saturated), 770 mg sodium
Eat this: *Baked potato with sour cream* 280 calories, 3 g fat (2 g saturated), 30 mg sodium	**Not that:** *Loaded baked potato* 620 calories, 31 g fat (19 g saturated), 570 mg sodium
Eat this: *Apple pie* 540 calories, 28 g fat (13 g saturated), 440 mg sodium	**Not that:** *Fudge cake or brownie sundae* 1130 calories, 57 g fat (30 g saturated), 400 mg sodium

Diner

ABS DIET ENDORSEMENTS:

Pot roast 370 calories, 16 g fat (7 g saturated), 570 mg sodium

Grilled chicken 476 calories, 14 g fat (3 g saturated), 1494 mg sodium

Vegetable of the day 60 calories, 3 g fat (1 g saturated), 150 mg sodium

THE LESSER OF TWO EVILS

Eat this: *Roast turkey with stuffing* 500 calories, 19 g fat (9 g saturated), 2190 mg sodium	**Not that:** *Chicken pot pie* 680 calories, 37 g fat (17 g saturated), 1590 mg sodium
Eat this: *Cole slaw* 170 calories, 14 g fat (2 g saturated), 380 mg sodium	**Not that:** *Fries* 600 calories, 30 g fat (12 g saturated), 460 mg sodium
Eat this: *Tuna melt* 537 calories, 28 g fat (13 g saturated), 1518 mg sodium	**Not that:** *Patty melt* 770 calories, 50 g fat (25 g saturated), 1130 mg sodium

Boston Market

ABS DIET ENDORSEMENTS:

Hand-carved rotisserie turkey 170 calories, 1 g fat (0 g saturated), 850 mg sodium

Fresh steamed broccoli 30 calories, 0 g fat (0 g saturated), 30 mg sodium

THE LESSER OF TWO EVILS

Eat this: *¼ sweet garlic rotisserie chicken (white meat, no skin or wing)* 170 calories, 4 g fat (1 g saturated), 480 mg sodium	**Not that:** *Chipotle meat loaf and chipotle gravy* 860 calories, 55 g fat (23 g saturated), 1750 mg sodium
Eat this: *Green beans* 70 calories, 4 g fat (0.5 g saturated), 250 mg sodium	**Not that:** *Squash casserole* 330 calories, 24 g fat (13 g saturated), 1110 mg sodium

Italian Restaurant (such as Olive Garden, Carrabba's, Macaroni Grill, or Fazoli's)

ABS DIET ENDORSEMENTS:

Minestrone soup (cup) 100 calories, 1 g fat (0 g saturated), 610 mg sodium

Chicken Marsala 460 calories, 25 g fat (7 g saturated), 790 mg sodium

THE LESSER OF TWO EVILS

Eat this: *Pasta with marinara sauce* 850 calories, 17 g fat (4 g saturated), 1450 mg sodium	**Not that:** *Pasta with Alfredo sauce* 1500 calories, 97 g fat (48 g saturated), 1030 mg sodium
Eat this: *Cheese ravioli with tomato sauce* 620 calories, 26 g fat (11 g saturated), 1290 mg sodium	**Not that:** *Lasagna* 960 calories, 53 g fat (21 g saturated), 2060 mg sodium
Eat this: *Soft breadsticks (2)* 280 calories, 12 g fat (2 g saturated), 640 mg sodium	**Not that:** *Antipasto (half an order)* 315 calories, 24 g fat (8 g saturated), 1480 mg sodium

Mexican Restaurant (such as Don Pablo's or Chili's)
ABS DIET ENDORSEMENTS:

Chicken fajitas with lettuce and pico de gallo 850 calories, 30 g fat (6 g saturated), 2100 mg sodium

Side of stewed black, kidney, or pinto beans 120 calories, 2 g fat (0 g saturated), 400 mg sodium

THE LESSER OF TWO EVILS

Eat this: *Enchiladas combo (beef and chicken)* 615 calories, 35 g fat (15 g saturated), 1800 mg sodium	**Not that:** *Chicken chimichanga* 1100 calories, 50 g fat (15 g saturated), 3300 mg sodium
Eat this: *Chips (12) with guacamole (2.5 ounces)* 380 calories, 22 g fat (4 g saturated), 300 mg sodium	**Not that:** *Chips (12) with cheese dip (2 ounces)* 440 calories, 25 g fat (7 g saturated), 920 mg sodium

Chinese Restaurant (such as Panda Express or P.F. Chang's)
ABS DIET ENDORSEMENTS:

Egg drop soup 60 calories, 3 g fat (1 g saturated), 1000 mg sodium

Stir-fried vegetables 750 calories, 19 g fat (3 g saturated), 2150 mg sodium

Szechuan shrimp 950 calories, 20 g fat (2 g saturated), 2460 mg sodium

THE LESSER OF TWO EVILS

Eat this: *Shrimp with garlic sauce* 950 calories, 30 g fat (4 g saturated), 2950 mg sodium	**Not that:** *Beef with broccoli* 1180 calories, 46 g fat (9 g saturated), 3150 mg sodium
Eat this: *Chicken chow mein* 1000 calories, 32 g fat (10 g saturated), 2450 mg sodium	**Not that:** *General Tso's chicken* 1600 calories, 60 g fat (10 g saturated), 3200 mg sodium
Eat this: *Vegetarian spring roll* 80 calories, 2.5 g fat (0 g saturated), 270 mg sodium	**Not that:** *Chicken/pork egg roll* 200 calories, 10 g fat (1 g saturated), 450 mg sodium

Sushi Bar

ABS DIET ENDORSEMENTS:

Edamame (2 ounces) 86 calories, 4 g fat (0 g saturated), 8 mg sodium

Miso soup (cup) 50 calories, 2 g fat (n/a g saturated), 310 mg sodium

Tuna roll (12 pieces) 260 calories, 1.5 g fat (0 g saturated), 270 mg sodium

Nigiri, salmon (3 pieces) 192 calories, 2 g fat (0 g saturated), 126 mg sodium

THE LESSER OF TWO EVILS

Eat this: *California roll (12 pieces)* 290 calories, 5 g fat (1 g saturated), 380 mg sodium	**Not that:** *Crunchy shrimp roll (12 pieces)* 650 calories, 19 g fat (2 g saturated), 1247 mg sodium
Eat this: *Nigiri, shrimp (3 pieces)* 267 calories, 2.5 g fat (0 g saturated), 273 mg sodium	**Not that:** *Nigiri, eel (3 pieces)* 258 calories, 7 g fat (1.5 g saturated), 432 mg sodium

Seafood Restaurant

ABS DIET ENDORSEMENTS:

Shrimp cocktail (3 ounces) 80 calories, 1 g fat (0 g saturated), 190 mg sodium

Grilled or broiled white fish (6 ounces) 210 calories, 5 g fat (1 g saturated), 360 mg sodium

Grilled or broiled salmon (8 ounces) 420 calories, 21 g fat (4 g saturated), 340 mg sodium

Salad with light dressing 90 calories, 7 g fat (1 g saturated), 490 mg sodium

THE LESSER OF TWO EVILS

Eat this: *Broiled salmon (8 ounces)* 420 calories, 21 g fat (4 g saturated), 340 mg sodium	**Not that:** *Fried white fish (9 ounces)* 520 calories, 24 g fat (8 g saturated), 840 mg sodium

THE LESSER OF TWO EVILS (CONT.)

Eat this: *Cup of Manhattan-style clam chowder* 153 calories, 1 g fat (0 g saturated), 680 mg sodium	**Not that:** *Cup of New England–style clam chowder* 250 calories, 7 g fat (2 g saturated), 1400 mg sodium

Pizza Places

Domino's

ABS DIET ENDORSEMENT:

2 slices medium thin-crust Vegi-Feast cheese pizza 336 calories, 19 g fat (7 g saturated), 793 mg sodium

THE LESSER OF TWO EVILS

Eat this: *2 slices medium thin-crust Hawaiian Feast pizza* 348 calories, 19 g fat (7 g saturated), 908 mg sodium	**Not that:** *2 slices medium hand-tossed Bacon Cheeseburger Feast pizza* 546 calories, 26 g fat (11 g saturated), 1268 mg sodium
Eat this: *Hot buffalo wings (2 pieces)* 90 calories, 5 g fat (1 g saturated), 508 mg sodium	**Not that:** *Cheesy Bread (2 pieces)* 246 calories, 13 g fat (4 saturated), 324 mg sodium

DANGER AT YOUR DOORSTEP

The TV ads are tempting, but which delivery pizza will turn your Blockbuster night into your very own *Return of the Blob*?

Domino's *2 slices medium (12") cheese pizza* 372 calories, 11 g fat (4 g saturated), 770 mg sodium

Little Caesar's *2 slices medium (12") round cheese pizza* 320 calories, 12 g fat (5 g saturated), 640 mg sodium

Pizza Hut *2 slices medium (12") hand-tossed crust cheese pizza* 480 calories, 16 g fat (9 g saturated), 1040 mg sodium

Papa John's *2 slices medium (12") original-crust cheese pizza* 420 calories, 16 g fat (5 g saturated), 1060 mg sodium

Pizza Hut
ABS DIET ENDORSEMENT:
2 slices medium Fit 'n' Delicious Ham, Pineapple, and Diced Tomato pizza 320 calories, 8 g fat (4 g saturated), 940 mg sodium

THE LESSER OF TWO EVILS

Eat this: *2 slices medium Thin 'n' Crispy Chicken Supreme pizza* 400 calories, 14 g fat (7 g saturated), 1040 mg sodium	**Not that:** *2 slices medium Pepperoni Lover's Pan pizza* 660 calories, 36 g fat (14 g saturated), 1340 mg sodium
Eat this: *Hot wings (2 pieces)* 110 calories, 6 g fat (2 g saturated), 450 mg sodium	**Not that:** *Cheese Breadsticks (2 pieces)* 400 calories, 20 g fat (7 g saturated), 680 mg sodium

Papa John's
ABS DIET ENDORSEMENT:
2 slices medium original-crust Garden Fresh pizza 380 calories, 12 g fat (3 g saturated), 940 mg sodium

THE LESSER OF TWO EVILS

Eat this: *2 slices medium original-crust Grilled Chicken Alfredo pizza* 420 calories, 14 g fat (5 g saturated), 1020 mg sodium	**Not that:** *2 slices medium original-crust The Meats pizza* 540 calories, 26 g fat (8 g saturated), 1420 mg sodium

DANGER IN YOUR FREEZER

Delivery pizza might seem like an extravagance when you could just pop one of those frozen pies into the oven, but ordering delivery can actually save you on calories and sodium as well. That's because pizza joints use mostly fresh ingredients. Here's a rundown of the most popular brands:

Tony's *2 slices cheese (Cut into ⅛ths)* 370 calories, 17 g fat (6 g saturated), 780 mg sodium

Freschetta *2 slices cheese (Cut into ⅛ths)* 463 calories, 16 g fat (7.5 g saturated), 1288 mg sodium

DiGiorno *2 slices cheese (Cut into ⅛ths)* 465 calories, 16.5 g fat (7.5 g saturated), 1275 mg sodium

THE LESSER OF TWO EVILS (CONT.)

Eat this: *Papa's Chicken Strips (2 pieces)* 160 calories, 8 g fat (2 g saturated), 350 mg sodium

Not that: *Cheesesticks (2 pieces)* 360 calories, 16 g fat (4.5 g saturated), 830 mg sodium

Smoothie Stands

I prefer you make your own smoothie, but sometimes you need one on the go. If so, always get yours with extra protein (you'd be surprised how many of these shakes are just fruit, water, and air). Then, make sure the shake contains a gram or two of fat, otherwise your body won't absorb many of the fat-soluble nutrients from all that fruit. Simply asking it to be made with low-fat milk or yogurt will do the trick. But beware fat bombs. Here's a clue: If it sounds more like a dessert than a beverage for someone with an active lifestyle, skip it.

Jamba Juice

ABS DIET ENDORSEMENTS:

Berry Fulfilling (16 ounces) 160 calories, 0.5 g fat (0 g saturated), 230 mg sodium

Orange Divine (16 ounces) 160 calories, 0.5 g fat (0 g saturated), 230 mg sodium

THE LESSER OF TWO EVILS

Eat this: *Banana Berry (16 ounces)* 310 calories, 0.5 g fat (0 g saturated), 75 mg sodium

Not that: *Chocolate Moo'd (16 ounces)* 500 calories, 6 g fat (4 g saturated), 260 mg sodium

Smoothie King

ABS DIET ENDORSEMENTS:

Slim-N-Trim vanilla 227 calories, 1 g fat (0 g saturated), 150 mg sodium

Blueberry Heaven 260 calories, 1 g fat (0 g saturated), 200 mg sodium

THE LESSER OF TWO EVILS

Eat this: *The Activator, Chocolate* 429 calories, 1 g fat (0 g saturated), 260 mg sodium	**Not that:** *Pina Colada Island* 550 calories, 11 g fat (9 g saturated), 300 mg sodium

Food Courts at Malls

Spend more time eating than you do shopping, and you'll end up having to go back—for bigger clothes. Don't even think about stopping at Cinnabon; eat one of their cinnamon-buns-on-steroids, and you'll rack up 813 calories and 8 grams of saturated fat. Here are the best stops so you won't drop while you shop.

Auntie Anne's

ABS DIET ENDORSEMENTS:

Jalapeño pretzel (without butter) with marinara sauce 280 calories, 1 g fat (0 g saturated), 960 mg sodium

Whole wheat pretzel (without butter) 350 calories, 1.5 g fat (0 g saturated), 1100 mg sodium

THE LESSER OF TWO EVILS

Eat this: *Garlic pretzel (without butter) with sweet mustard* 380 calories, 2.5 g fat (1 g saturated), 950 mg sodium	**Not that:** *Original pretzel (without butter) with cheese sauce* 440 calories, 9 g fat (4 g saturated), 1410 mg sodium

Mrs. Fields

ABS DIET ENDORSEMENT:

Debra's Special Nibbler Cookie 100 calories, 4.5 g fat (2 g saturated), 80 mg sodium

THE LESSER OF TWO EVILS

Eat this: *Peanut Butter Bite-Size Nibbler Cookie* 110 calories, 6 g fat (2.5 g saturated), 95 mg sodium	**Not that:** *Milk Chocolate Chip Cookie* 280 calories, 13 g fat (8 g saturated), 180 mg sodium

Sbarro

ABS DIET ENDORSEMENTS:

1 slice fresh tomato pizza 450 calories, 14 g fat (n/a g saturated), 1040 mg sodium

1 slice mushroom pizza 460 calories, 14 g fat (n/a g saturated), 1310 mg sodium

Greek salad (side) 60 calories, 5 g fat (n/a g saturated), 130 mg sodium

THE LESSER OF TWO EVILS

Eat this: *1 slice chicken vegetable pizza* 530 calories, 17 g fat (n/a g saturated), 1260 mg sodium	**Not that:** *1 slice pepperoni pizza* 730 calories, 37 g fat (n/a g saturated), 2200 mg sodium

Ballparks

I'm a big fan of smuggling in your own food: It makes healthy eating easier, it makes you feel like a little bit of a rebel, and it avoids the humiliation of paying $453 for one hot dog. But if you can't or won't smuggle trail mix in your underwear, you can still grab a handful of Powerfoods. If you have to pile something on, make it insults to the other team, not nacho cheese.

ABS DIET ENDORSEMENTS:

Roasted peanuts in shell, unsalted (3 ounces) 510 calories, 37 g fat (7.5 g saturated), 0 mg sodium

Light beer (12 ounces) 103 calories, 0 g fat (0 g saturated), 0 mg sodium

THE LESSER OF TWO EVILS

Eat this: *Nachos (12–16 nachos)* 692 calories, 38 g fat (16 g saturated), 1632 mg sodium	**Not that:** *Popcorn popped in oil (medium, 16-cup serving)* 880 calories, 50 g fat (9 g saturated), 1556 mg sodium

THE LESSER OF TWO EVILS (CONT.)

Eat this: *Regular beer (12 ounces)* 139 calories, 0 g fat (0 g saturated), 14 mg sodium	**Not that:** *Cola (16 ounces)* 155 calories, 0 g fat (0 g saturated), 15 mg sodium

Sports Bars

Alcohol will weaken your defenses; so will the fact that 380-pound offensive tackles are considered pro athletes. So I'll make you a deal: If you are paid millions of dollars to shove enormous men in helmets each Sunday, then order whatever you want. If not, then follow the guidelines below.

ABS DIET ENDORSEMENT:

Salted nuts (per ounce) 168 calories, 15 g fat (2 g saturated), 190 mg sodium

Hot wings (4–5 wings) 350 calories, 24 g fat (8 g saturated), 510 mg sodium

Fried mozzarella sticks (3 pieces) 375 calories, 21 g fat (7 saturated), 780 mg sodium

THE LESSER OF TWO EVILS

Eat this: *Chicken fingers (5 pieces)* 620 calories, 34 g fat (13 g saturated), 1450 mg sodium	**Not that:** *Cheese fries with ranch dressing (2 cups)* 1500 calories, 108 g fat (46 g saturated), 1300 mg sodium
Eat this: *Burger (Lettuce, tomato, onion, mustard)* 660 calories, 36 g fat (17 g saturated), 810 mg sodium	**Not that:** *Mushroom cheeseburger* 900 calories, 57 g fat (28 g saturated), 1070 mg sodium

Ice Cream Shops

First, come here directly after a meal. You'll be less likely to pig out. Second, don't stress too much about it; ice cream may be sugary and high in calories, but it also provides protein and calcium.

As indulgences go, it's hardly a high crime. So don't waste your time on nasty no-sugar-added ice creams; no sense eating food you don't enjoy. Instead, look for reduced-fat options and add Powerfoods (nuts and fruit) whenever possible. And if you completely ignore all that advice, take this tip: Order the ice cream you absolutely love . . . in a single-scoop cup.

Baskin-Robbins

ABS DIET ENDORSEMENTS:

Espresso 'n Cream low-fat ice cream (1 scoop) 180 calories, 4 g fat (1.5 g saturated), 120 mg sodium

Perils of Praline low-fat yogurt (1 scoop) 190 calories, 3.5 g fat (1.5 g saturated), 170 mg sodium

THE LESSER OF TWO EVILS

Eat this: *Very Berry Strawberry ice cream (1 scoop)* 220 calories, 11 g fat (7 g saturated), 70 mg sodium	**Not that:** *Fudge Brownie ice cream (2 scoops)* 600 calories, 38 g fat (22 g saturated), 280 mg sodium

Cold Stone Creamery

ABS DIET ENDORSEMENT:

Low-fat chocolate ice cream with blueberries or strawberries ("Like it" size) 240 calories, 1.5 g fat (1 g saturated), 140 mg sodium

THE LESSER OF TWO EVILS

Eat this: *Any fruit-flavored ice cream (strawberry, raspberry, banana, etc.) with blueberries ("Like it" size)* 210 calories, 22 g fat (14 g saturated), 90 mg sodium	**Not that:** *Any fruit-flavored ice cream (strawberry, raspberry, banana, etc.) with brownie pieces in a cone ("Love it" size)* 670 calories, 46 g fat (26 g saturated), 400 mg sodium

HE WANTED TO CHASE AFTER HIS KIDS, SO HE CHASED AFTER A GOAL

Name: William Salerno

Age: 38

Height: 5'9"

Weight, Week 1: 222

Weight, Week 6: 198

Having twins 2 years ago meant that William Salerno was going to be busier than ever. He was in a job that required him to routinely work 12-hour days, plus now he had to help care for two young children. And that's when it hit him.

"I feel like I'm an older dad and that I gotta stay ahead of these guys," Salerno says. "I want to be like my father was with me—always active. And that got me thinking."

That's when his business manager told him he had to read *The Abs Diet*.

"When I read it, something clicked. I'm amazed by it because I usually don't go for those kinds of books. Usually they don't do anything for me," he says. "I started to read it in my office one day and read it for a couple hours. I carried it everywhere. Now I talk about trans fats and high-fructose corn syrup to anybody who'll listen to me."

He reads food ingredients on everything—and remains pumped up about the plan.

"Almonds are a god," he says.

A side benefit is that he no longer experiences any symptoms with gout—a disorder that causes pain in the joints that's hampered Salerno in the past.

"My theory is that if I'm 220, then I could very well have been 230—I was in that range for a couple of years," Salerno says. "People see me now and they say, where'd it all go? They think I'm starving myself, and I'm not. It's so refreshing and unbelievable."

Now, he can't stop talking about it.

"I quoted passages to my wife so often that she began calling me 'the *Abs Diet* zealot.'"

Chapter 10

INDULGE AND ENJOY

The Abs Diet Holiday Survival Guide

IF A DIET IS AN ANT, then the holidays are the bottom of a shoe, because they have the power to squash you every time. Between the cookies, meat loaf, more cookies, eggnog, fruitcake, mashed potatoes and gravy (oh, the gravy), many of us cram 6 months of eating into 6 weeks. The result: Come January, the only thing you're trying to cram is 4 extra inches into your jeans.

As you know, the Abs Diet isn't about deprivation, so I want you to have the occasional tussle with a kilo-high mound of stuffing. If you do that for 6 weeks straight, you'll have succeeded—on the Flabs Diet. Since you have one cheat meal per week, I suggest you play your card around the biggest bomb—whether it's Thanksgiving dinner, the Christmas party, or a date with Aunt Matilda's can't-resist chocolate cheesecake—and then sidestep the dietary land mines through the rest of the week. To eat right throughout the holidays, these choices will help you avoid turning your diet into a disaster.

Halloween
THE LESSER OF TWO EVILS

Eat this: *Bit-O-Honey*

Per 6 pieces: 186 calories, 4 g fat (0 g saturated), 124 mg sodium

Not that: *Whoppers*

Per 9 pieces: 125 calories, 7 g fat (4 g saturated), 38 mg sodium

---

Eat this: *Kit Kat*

Per miniature bar: 51 calories, 3 g fat (1.7 g saturated), 6 mg sodium

Not that: *Reese's Pieces*

About 30 pieces: 120 calories, 6 g fat (4 g saturated), 47 mg sodium

---

Eat this: *Milky Way*

Per fun-size piece: 76 calories, 3 g fat (1 g saturated), 43 mg sodium

Not that: *Butterfinger*

Per fun-size piece: 100 calories, 4 g fat (2 g saturated), 45 mg sodium

---

Thanksgiving Dinner
THE LESSER OF TWO EVILS

Eat this: *1 serving turkey breast*

²⁄₃ cup mashed potatoes

¹⁄₃ cup turkey gravy

1 dinner roll

1 cup corn

1 slice jellied cranberry sauce

1 slice pumpkin pie

TOTAL: 1233 calories, 39 g fat (11 g saturated), 1493 mg sodium

Not that: *1 serving dark turkey meat*

1 cup stuffing

²⁄₃ cup sweet potatoes with marsh-mallow topping

1 cup green-bean casserole

1 cup homemade cranberry sauce

1 slice pecan pie

TOTAL: 1944 calories, 90 g fat (26 g saturated), 2512 mg sodium

---

Thanksgiving Leftovers
THE LESSER OF TWO EVILS

Eat this: *1 serving turkey breast on 2 pieces whole grain bread with let-tuce, cranberry sauce*

½ cup green-bean casserole

TOTAL: 530 calories, 20 g fat (7 g saturated), 1015 mg sodium

Not that: *1 serving turkey on kaiser roll with mayo*

²⁄₃ cup mashed potatoes

¹⁄₃ cup turkey gravy

TOTAL: 665 calories, 30 g fat (7 g saturated), 1300 mg sodium

Black Friday at the Mall

THE LESSER OF TWO EVILS

Eat this: *1 Auntie Anne's Cinnamon-Sugar pretzel (without butter)* 350 calories, 2 g fat (0 g saturated), 430 mg sodium

Not that: *1 Cinnabon cinnamon bun* 813 calories, 32 g fat (8 g saturated, 5 g trans fat), 801 mg sodium

Eat this: *TCBY frozen yogurt (small)* 110 calories, 0 g fat, 60 mg sodium

Not that: *Orange Julius (small)* 220 calories, 1 g fat (0 g saturated), 10 mg sodium

At the Office in December

THE LESSER OF TWO EVILS

Eat this: *1 handful roasted pistachios* 175 calories, 14 g fat (1.7 g saturated), 125 mg sodium

Not that: *1 handful (¼ cup) holiday M&M's* 256 calories, 11 g fat (7 g saturated), 32 mg sodium

Eat this: *1 brownie (2" square)* 165 calories, 7 g fat (2 g saturated), 82 mg sodium

Not that: *A few chunks of peanut brittle* 274 calories, 11 g fat (2 g saturated), 252 mg sodium

Eat this: *1 Hershey's Kiss* 26 calories, 1.5 g fat (1 g saturated), 4 mg sodium

Not that: *1 1-ounce candy cane* 110 calories, 0 g fat, 11 mg sodium

Christmas Dinner
THE LESSER OF TWO EVILS

Eat this: *8 ounces turkey breast*	**Not that:** *8 ounces ham*
⅔ cup stuffing	*Dinner roll with 2 pats butter*
1 cup sweet potatoes	*1 cup mashed potatoes*
1 slice cranberry sauce	*½ cup gravy*
⅔ cup creamed corn	*1 cup green-bean casserole*
Sliver pecan pie	*Slice pumpkin pie with heavy*
Sliver pumpkin pie	*whipped cream*
Glass of red wine	*Glass of beer*
TOTAL: 1653 calories, 50 g fat (12 g saturated), 1444 mg sodium	TOTAL: 1670 calories, 87 g fat (41 g saturated), 5671 mg sodium

New Year's Eve
THE LESSER OF TWO EVILS

Eat this: *12 large shrimp with 2 tablespoons cocktail sauce* 125 calories, 1 g fat (0 g saturated), 948 mg sodium	**Not that:** *1 small crab cake* 285 calories, 12 g fat (2 g saturated), 807 mg sodium
Drink this: *Champagne* 105 calories, 0 g fat, 0 mg sodium	**Not that:** *Vodka tonic* 125 calories, 0 g fat, 7 mg sodium
Eat this: *8 melon balls wrapped in prosciutto* 220 calories, 11 g fat (4 g saturated), 1650 mg sodium	**Not that:** *1 potato pancake with smoked salmon and caviar* 313 calories, 17 g fat (4 g saturated), 1760 mg sodium

Feasts, Not Famine

At the end of the year, you're tempted everywhere—at meals, at the secretary's candy jar, under the mistletoe. If you can make it through the biggest fat wave of the year, the other 10 months will be smoother than a supermodel's freshly shaved legs. Sure, you'll hit the occasional holiday feast. Go ahead and enjoy them, but know that you can always make decisions to satisfy your tastes and cravings without drowning yourself in fat.

Super Bowl Party

THE LESSER OF TWO EVILS

Eat this: *2 handfuls assorted nuts*	**Not that:** *Celery with onion dip*
Baked tortilla chips with salsa	*Nacho chips with 7-layer bean and cheese dip*
2 slices turkey or roast beef hoagie with cheese	*15 hot wings*
TOTAL: 848 calories, 36 g fat (10 g saturated), 2372 mg sodium	TOTAL:1264 calories, 86 g fat (26 g saturated), 2229 mg sodium

St. Patrick's Day

THE LESSER OF TWO EVILS

Drink this: *Guinness (12 ounces)* 126 calories; *Beamish Irish Crème Stout (12 ounces)* 146 calories; *Amstel Light (12 ounces)* 99 calories	**Not that:** *Beck's Dark (12 ounces)* 146 calories; *Sam Adams Cream Stout (12 ounces)* 195 calories; *Michelob Light (12 ounces)* 134 calories

Easter Dinner

THE LESSER OF TWO EVILS

Eat this: *1 8-ounce serving lamb*	**Not that:** *1 8-ounce serving ham*
1 cup roasted potatoes with olive oil	*1 cup potato salad*
1 cup steamed spinach	*1 cup corn*
Salad with oil and balsamic vinegar	*Caesar salad with Caesar dressing*
TOTAL: 958 calories, 64 g fat (18 g saturated), 502 mg sodium	TOTAL: 1245 calories, 72 g fat (18 g saturated), 1818 mg sodium

Easter Basket

THE LESSER OF TWO EVILS

Eat this: *Jelly beans (about 20 pieces)* 82 calories, 0 g fat, 11 mg sodium	**Not that:** *Werther's Original* Per 6 pieces: 120 calories, 2 g fat (2 g saturated fat), 120 mg sodium
Eat this: *2 marshmallow peeps* 64 calories, 0 g fat, 6 mg sodium	**Not that:** *1 Cadbury Crème Egg* 170 calories, 6 g fat (3.5 g saturated), 25 mg sodium

Fourth of July

THE LESSER OF TWO EVILS

Eat this: *1 quarter-pound grilled burger with ketchup, mustard, lettuce, tomato, slice of cheese* *1 cup homemade coleslaw* TOTAL: 548 calories, 24 g fat (9 g saturated), 806 mg sodium	**Not that:** *2 fried chicken legs* *½ cup macaroni salad* TOTAL: 1093 calories, 70 g fat (16 g saturated), 1061 mg sodium

Chapter 11

CRANK UP THE FAT BURN

The Abs Diet Workout

BETWEEN YOUR JOB, family, home, and Google addiction, you probably feel pushed and pulled in more directions than a piece of Silly Putty. Me, too.

The clock seems to move faster and faster, and we're all running to keep up. We crave less stress, more time, and 30 uninterrupted seconds during which nobody nags us about meeting deadlines, caulking cracks, or playing a 14th consecutive game of Candy Land.

We're all busy. But we're not too busy to exercise.

Here's the proof: The average American spends 28 hours a week watching television. If you watch only one-half as much TV, that still means you have more than a solid half a day of quality time you're spending with O'Reilly, the Donald, or the Three Stooges (Simon, Paula, and Randy) every week.

Give up just one of those hours each week—just one—and you can change your body and your life forever.

I said at the very beginning of this book that the Abs Diet was no ordinary diet, and I meant it. To me, one of the biggest errors in most mainstream diets is that they treat exercise the way the prom queen treats the chess champ—with indifference. They operate on ho-hum exercise principles: Great if you do it, so what if you don't.

But most plans overlook one simple truth: The best way to lose fat is to build muscle and let that muscle eat away flab from the inside out. Each pound of muscle you build means your body will burn an extra up to 50 calories a day just sitting still. Add 5 pounds of muscle—something you can easily do over the course of 6 weeks—and you're now burning an extra up to 1,750 calories a week! When it comes down to it, exercise can do just as much to reshape your body as any broccoli floret can.

Of course, the ABS DIET POWER 12 gives you all the weapons you need to fight fat: protein, healthy fat, whole grains, and fiber to keep you full, to feed your body nutrients, and to ward off potentially devastating hunger pangs. But you'll accelerate all of your gains with the secret weapon in your dietary artillery: muscle.

I'm not talking bar-bouncer, piano-lifting muscle. I'm talking about lean muscle mass, which works as your body's natural metabolism booster. To make the Abs Diet as effective as possible, you need to add a muscle-building and strength-training workout to your program.

Now, if the only dumbbells you know live four doors down, then the prospect of taking up strength training may seem intimidating. It shouldn't be. Like the Abs Diet itself, the Abs Diet Workout is designed to be fast, simple, effective, and convenient. I know you're not going to spend hours a day in the gym, I know you're not going to enjoy a workout program that's all pain and no gain, and I know you're not going to stick with it if you don't see impressive results, fast. That's why I've created a workout program that will build muscle, melt away fat, and reintroduce you to your abs—all in just 20 minutes a day, 3 days a week.

How do I know it works? Besides the countless success stories of people who reshaped their bodies with minimal time at the gym, one study found that you can put on 6 pounds of muscle and lose 15 pounds of fat in 6 weeks by following the exercise principles used in the Abs Diet Workout. We're talking just 20 minutes a day, just 3 days a week.

Don't believe it? Think you need to quit your job and spend your life in the gym to see results? Well, check this out: Scientists at the University of Glamorgan in Wales studied 16 weight lifters doing either one or three sets of upper-body exercises three times a week. Those who did one set gained just as much muscle—and burned twice as much fat—as the three-set group. In other words, the less time you spend, the better your results!

What's great about this program is that you can do it in a gym or in your house, you don't need fancy equipment, and you can finish it before *ER* is even halfway over. (In fact, I've even included a no-weight workout that you can do in your backyard, in a hotel room, in a prison cell if need be. No excuses, remember?) One hour a week. That's all I want, and that's all you need.

Your 3-Days-a-Week Muscle-Building, Fat-Burning Program

Think of muscle as your body's python and fat as a quivering mouse. In the battle between the two, the python will always win. And the bigger your python, the more mice it eats.

What's great about weight training is that it burns fat in three ways. First, there are the calories you burn off breaking a sweat. Second, there's the fact that new muscle eats up calories, making your body more efficient at burning fat. And third, there's the "afterburn"—the additional calories burned off in the hours immediately following your workout. All kinds of exercise raise your metabolism and give you an afterburn. But the effects of weight training far outstrip those of aerobic exercise. In one study, researchers found that the increased calorie burn of aerobics (that is, steady-state cardiovascular exercise like running or cycling) lasted only 30 minutes to an hour after a workout. In subjects who trained with weights, the increased metabolism lasted as long as 48 hours. That's 2 days during which your body burns fat after the fact.

And you don't need to push iron like a Nebraska offensive tackle to achieve the afterburn effect. All you have to do is employ the two major Abs Diet components of muscle building: circuit training and compound exercises.

Circuit training. There are many different ways to lift weights. A lot of people employ the lift-rest-lift-rest approach to weight training, and that's fine. But my guess is that you're interested in building the most muscle and burning the most fat in the least amount of time possible. So I've built the Abs Diet Workout around circuit training. In this type of training, there is no rest phase, no part of the workout where you're standing around the water fountain looking lost. Circuit training means that your body is constantly working, constantly improving.

BONUS: ADVANCED ABS!

If you're starting to feel as if your abs are tighter than the jeans you just pulled out of the dryer, then you're probably ready for a more challenging abdominal exercise. Try this one. Lie on your back on a Swiss ball, with your knees bent at 90 degrees, your feet flat, and your hands behind your ears. Keeping your right foot planted, lift your left foot off the floor and bring it toward you as you curl your torso up and to the left so that you right elbow meets your left knee. It's like the classic bicycle maneuver, and it works your entire core at once. Do 12 repetitions. Then plant your left foot on the floor and curl toward your right knee for another 12 reps.

Simply put, circuit training involves moving from one exercise to the next with little rest in between. Once you complete the circuit of 9 or 11 exercises, you rest for 2 minutes and then start again. In your time-compressed life, circuit training works because it means you're working the most muscles in the least amount of time; plus, with little rest, your heart rate stays elevated to give you an additional calorie burn. A recent Ohio University study found that a short-but-hard workout was effective in burning fat. Using a circuit of three exercises in a row for 31 minutes, the subjects were still burning more calories than normal 38 hours after the workout.

Compound exercises. Just like compound interest, compound exercises give you more back than you put in. Compound exercises hit many muscles during a single move (the squat engages 256 muscles at once!), so that you're gaining the most benefit from your workout. Compound exercises also ensure that you work the largest muscles in your body (like your chest, legs, and back). Larger muscles take more calories to maintain than smaller ones, making your workout that much more effective.

To put it all together, all you need is a gym membership or, if you're exercising at home, a set of dumbbells and a bench. (For dumbbells, I recommend you invest in an adjustable pair so that you can change weights for different exercises and up the resistance as you grow stronger.) Though it doesn't matter where you do the circuit, it does matter when you do it. Stick to 3 days a week with at least 1 day a week of rest in between to allow your muscles to recover and grow.

The Abs Diet Circuit

Perform each exercise once, then move immediately to the next exercise with only 30 seconds of rest in between. When you reach the end of the circuit, rest for 2 minutes and then repeat. Beginners can start with light weights and one circuit. More advanced lifters can do two or three circuits with weights that they can comfortably handle for at least 8 repetitions but no more than 12 repetitions.

ULTIMATE NO-WEIGHT WORKOUT

Sometimes, you can't get to the gym or even access the workout gear you have stashed in your basement. Maybe you're stuck in some godforsaken Motel 6. Maybe you're trapped at your in-laws' house. Maybe the Feds discovered you gave stock advice to Martha Stewart. Well, that's still no excuse. This full-body routine requires no equipment and only 8 minutes of your time. Perform each exercise below for 30 seconds. Do one move after another without rest and repeat the sequence without rest for a total of four times, if you can.

The intensity of this workout conditions your muscular and cardiovascular systems, helps improve flexibility, and melts fat. You'll burn hundreds of calories.

Jumping Jack. Just like grade school. Start with your hands on your hips and your feet together. Raise your hands out to your sides and up overhead as you move your feet out to the sides. Then bring your feet back together and lower your hands to your sides.

Split Hop. Stand with your hands on your hips and your feet together. Move your left foot 6 inches forward and your right foot 6 inches back. Now jump up and switch leg positions so that your right foot is forward.

Squat Thrust with Pushup. Stand with your arms at your sides. Bend your knees and lower your hands to the floor. Kick your legs behind you so that you're in a Pushup position. Now do a Pushup. Thrust your knees to your chest so that your feet are back underneath you and stand back up.

Mountain Climber. Get back in the Pushup position and kick your knees to your chest, one leg at a time. Alternate thrusting your knees forward, like you're running, so that one leg is extended when one knee is forward.

EXERCISE	REPETITIONS	REST	SETS
Squat	10–12	30 seconds	2
Bench Press	10	30 seconds	2
Pulldown	10	30 seconds	2
Military Press	10	30 seconds	2
Upright Row	10	30 seconds	2
Triceps Pushdown	10–12	30 seconds	2
Leg Extension	10–12	30 seconds	2
Biceps Curl	10	30 seconds	2
Leg Curl	10–12	30 seconds	2

Note: One day a week, add the following two exercises (do the Traveling Lunge after the Pulldown, and the Step-Up after the Upright Row). Because your legs contain your body's largest muscles, the fat-burning potential increases with a little extra time spent working your legs muscles.

EXERCISE	REPETITIONS	REST	SETS
Traveling Lunge	10–12 (each leg)	30 seconds	2
Step-Up	10–12 (each leg)	30 seconds	2

Squat. Hold a barbell with an overhand grip so that it rests comfortably on your upper back. Set your feet shoulder width apart, and keep your knees slightly bent, back straight, and eyes focused straight ahead. Slowly lower your body as if you were sitting back into a chair, keeping your back in its natural alignment and your lower legs perpendicular to the floor. When your thighs are parallel to the floor, pause, then return to the starting position.

Home variation: Same, but with one dumbbell in each hand, your palms facing your outer thighs.

Bench Press. Lie on your back on a flat bench with your feet on the floor. Grab the barbell with an overhand grip, your hands just beyond shoulder width apart. Lift the bar off the uprights, and hold it at arm's length over your chest. Slowly lower the bar to your chest. Pause, then push the bar back to the starting position.

Home variation: Pushups. Get in a Pushup position with your hands shoulder width apart. Bend at the elbows while keeping your back straight, until your chin almost touches the floor, then push back up.

Pulldown. Stand facing a lat pulldown machine. Reach up and grasp the bar with an overhand grip that's 4 to 6 inches wider than your shoulders. Sit on the seat, letting the resistance of the bar extend your arms above your head. When you're in position, pull the bar down until it touches your upper chest. Hold the position for a second, then return to the starting position.

Home variation: Bent-Over Row. Stand with your knees slightly bent and shoulder width apart. Bend over so that your back is almost parallel to the floor. Holding a dumbbell in each hand, let your arms hang toward the floor. With your palms facing in, pull the dumbbells toward you until they touch the outside of your chest. Pause, then return to the starting position.

Military Press. Sitting on an exercise bench, hold a barbell at shoulder height with your hands shoulder width apart. Press the weight straight overhead so that your arms are almost fully extended, hold for a count of one, then bring it down to the front of your shoulders.

Home variation: Sitting on a sturdy chair instead of a bench, hold one dumbbell in each hand, about level with your ears. Push the dumbbells straight overhead so that your arms are almost fully extended, hold for a count of one, then return to the starting position.

Upright Row. Grab a barbell with an overhand grip and stand with your feet shoulder width apart and your knees slightly bent. Let the barbell hang at arm's length on top of your thighs, thumbs pointed toward each other. Bending your elbows, lift your upper arms straight out to the sides, and pull the barbell straight up until your upper arms are parallel to the floor and the bar is just below chin level. Pause, then return to the starting position.

Home variation: Same, using one dumbbell in each hand.

Triceps Pushdown. While standing, grip a bar attached to a high pulley cable or lat machine with your hands 6 inches apart. With your elbows tucked against your sides, bring the bar down until it is directly in front of you. With your forearms parallel to the floor (the starting position), push the bar down until your arms are extended straight down with the bar near your thigh. Don't lock your elbows. Return to the starting position.

Home variation: Triceps Kickback. Holding a light dumbbell in each hand, stand with your knees slightly bent and shoulder width apart. Bend over so that your back is almost parallel to the ground. Bend your elbows to about 90-degree angles, raising them to just above the level of your back. This is the starting position. Extend your forearms backward, keeping your upper arms stationary. When they're fully extended, your arms should be parallel to the ground. Pause, then return to the starting position.

WHAT'S MY MOTIVATION?

No matter how dedicated you are to your weight-loss goals, there are some days when you don't feel like getting out of bed, much less getting to the gym. How do you keep making progress? Here are a few tricks to keep you from falling off the exercise wagon.

Make a bet. Challenge a coworker to a contest—the first to drop 10 pounds, best of seven in one-on-one, and so forth. Competition is the ultimate motivator.

Switch training partners. Working out with a partner who will hold you accountable for showing up at the gym works well—for a while. But the longer you know him, the easier it is to back out of a workout. Find a new one every few months.

Strike an agreement with your family. The rule: You get 1 hour to yourself every day, provided that you use it for exercise (and reciprocate the favor).

Schedule a body-composition test every 2 months. The short-term end date will keep you focused to keep moving forward.

Leg Extension. Sitting on a leg extension machine with your feet under the footpads, lean back slightly, and lift the pads with your feet until your legs are extended.

Home variation: Stand with your back flat against a wall. Squat down so that your thighs are parallel to the ground. Hold that position for as long as you can. That consists of one set. Aim for 20 seconds to start and work your way up to 45 seconds.

Biceps Curl. Stand while holding a barbell in front of you, palms facing out, with your hands shoulder width apart and your arms hanging in front of you. Curl the weight toward your shoulders, hold for a second, then return to the starting position.

Home variation: Same, only use a set of dumbbells instead.

Leg Curl. Lie facedown on a leg curl machine and hook your ankles under the padded bar. Keeping your stomach and pelvis against the bench, slowly raise your feet toward your butt, curling up the weight. Come up so that your feet nearly touch your butt, and slowly return to the starting position.

Home variation: Lie down with your stomach on the floor. Put a light dumbbell between your feet (so that the top end of the dumbbell rests on the bottom of your feet). Squeeze your feet together and curl them up toward your butt.

Traveling Lunge. Rest a barbell against your upper back. Stand, with your feet hip width apart, at one end of the room; you need room to walk about 20 steps. Step forward with your left foot, and lower your body so that your left thigh is parallel to the floor and your right thigh is perpendicular to the floor (your right knee should bend and almost touch the floor). Stand and bring your right foot up next to your left, then repeat with the right leg lunging forward.

Home variation: Use dumbbells, holding one in each hand with your arms at your sides. If you don't have enough space, do the move in one place, alternating your lead foot with each lunge.

Step-Up. Use a step or bench that's 18 inches off the ground. Place your left foot on the step so that your knee is bent at 90 degrees. Your knee should not advance past the toes of your left foot. Push off with your left foot and bring your right foot onto the step, keeping your back straight. Now step down with the left foot, followed by the right. Alternate the leading foot, or do all of the repetitions leading with one foot and then alternating. Once you're comfortable, add dumbbells.

Home variation: Same, only use a staircase instead of a step (if you don't have one).

Abdominal Exercises: Before Your Circuit

You'd think with a name like the Abs Diet, I'd be asking you to spend more time working your abs than J.Lo spends working the counters at Tiffany & Co. But finding your abs isn't as much about abdominal exercises as it is about changing your body composition to eliminate the belly fat that's covering them. Once you do that, then you can concentrate on building the muscle. It's sort of like a construction company trying to build a housing development. If you don't clear the lot of sand, debris, and trees, you aren't going to have any room to build the house. But if you clear the lot and lay the foundation, then you can build a house that everyone will see.

To work your abs, you'll want to hit all five parts of your abdominal region (as outlined below). At the beginning of your strength circuit (2 or 3 days a week), do these five exercises in a circuit with little rest in between each. Start with one set, but work up to doing two or three sets. To vary your exercises, see *The Abs Diet,* which has 50 variations of abdominal moves.

Traditional Crunch (works the upper part of the rectus abdominis, which is the six-pack muscle that helps you maintain good posture). Lie on your back with your knees bent and your hands behind your ears. Slowly crunch up, bringing your shoulder blades off the ground. Do 12 to 15 repetitions.

Flutter Kick (works the lower part of the rectus abdominis).

Lie on your back, raise both feet off the ground, and scissor-kick one leg over the other. Do 20 repetitions.

Saxon Side Bend (works the external and internal obliques, which extend diagonally down the sides of your waist and rotate the torso). Hold a pair of lightweight dumbbells over your head, in line with your shoulders, with your elbows slightly bent. Keep your back straight, and slowly bend directly to your left side as far as possible without twisting your upper body. Pause, return to an upright position, then bend to your right side as far as possible. Do 6 to 10 repetitions.

Bridge (works the transverse abdominis, which is known as the girdle because it compresses the abdomen). Start to get in a Pushup position, but bend your elbows and rest your weight on your forearms instead. Your body should form a straight line. Pull your abdominals in. Hold for 20 seconds, breathing steadily. Do 1 to 2 repetitions.

Superman (works the lower back, which anchors all of the abdominal muscles). Lie with your stomach on the ground and your arms in front of you and legs behind you (in Superman-flying position). Lift your arms and legs about 6 inches off the ground and hold for as long as you can. Repeat three times.

Interval Training: 1 Day a Week

Back in the '80s, the only thing more popular than big hair and shoulder pads was running. Weight-loss experts touted long, steady aerobic exercise as nearly the best way to burn fat, build endurance, and keep the heart pumping.

And aerobic exercise (running, cycling, swimming) is good for you. I've run the New York City Marathon twice myself, and I can attest to the fact that cardiovascular exercise strengthens your heart, burns calories, and decreases stress.

But cardio has two significant drawbacks. First, it only burns calories while you're doing it, not afterward. And second, it does nothing to build muscle. Unless . . . unless you try interval training.

Interval training refers to a shorter, more intense method of working out. Instead of long, slow, boring runs or rides, interval training intersperses short bursts of high-intensity exertion with periods of slow, more restful exercise. In a Canadian study from Laval University, researchers measured differences in fat loss between two groups of exercisers following two different workout programs. The first group rode stationary bikes at a steady pace four or five times a week and burned 300 to 400 calories per 30- to 45-minute session. The second group did the same, but only one or two times a week, and they filled the rest of their sessions with short intervals of high-intensity cycling. They hopped on their stationary bikes and pedaled as quickly as they could for 30 to 90 sec-

ULTIMATE TOTAL-BODY DUMBBELL EXERCISE

Dumbbells are one of the smartest fitness investments you can make. They're portable and affordable, and they condition your body even more effectively than standard barbells, because they teach your body to balance and allow for a greater range of motion.

I've created here a super-simple, super-fast dumbbell workout that will hit your whole body at once. Do one set of 12 repetitions, and you're set for the day.

▶ Grab a pair of light dumbbells and get into a Pushup position, with your arms straight and directly beneath your shoulders.

▶ Do a Pushup. Then bring your feet underneath you, one foot at a time.

▶ Keeping your back flat, stand up. (This is a deadlift.)

▶ From the standing position, curl the weights up to your shoulders.

▶ Swing your elbows out to your sides so that the weights are above your shoulders.

▶ Lower your body until your thighs are parallel to the floor. Pause, then stand up as you press the weights overhead.

onds, rested, and then repeated the process several times per exercise session. As a result, they burned 225 to 250 calories while cycling, but they burned more fat at the end of the study than the workers in group one. In fact, even though they exercised less,

ABS DIET SUCCESS STORY

MORE ENERGY TO WORK, TO PLAY, AND TO CARE FOR HIS FAMILY

Name: Pete Hemmer

Age: 40

Weight, Week 1: 244

Weight, Week 6: 231

Weight, Week 10: 217

Pete Hemmer knew he had to get his body back in order. He had reached 286 pounds and was trying to care for premature triplets. He was unhappy—and out of shape, out of breath, out of energy. "When I stepped on the scale and saw 286, I said at that moment, 'I'm going to be 300 pounds. If I keep going where I'm going, I'll be dead by the time I'm 40,'" he says. That's when he knew he needed to change, so he just tried adjusting portion sizes and making smart choices about eating. Over the course of about a year and a half, he whittled himself down to 244 pounds—still far off from where he wanted to be. Then he read about the Abs Diet and told his wife, Krista, "That's the diet plan I need.

"I went out that weekend and bought the book, read it in a weekend from cover to cover, and my wife said I wouldn't shut up talking about it," he says. Then Krista asked him if it was something she could try, too. On Monday, they made their plan, and on Tuesday, they started.

"As I was pushing the cart down the aisle, I noticed there weren't any boxes in my cart. It was fresh vegetables, dairy and meat, and there were no frozen pizzas. All the stuff that had becomes staples of our their fat loss was nine times greater. Researchers said that the majority of the fat-burning took place after the workout.

So instead of asking you to spend 30 minutes on a stairclimber or a stationary bike every day, I want you to add one simple inter-

diet were missing," he says. "It was just something that struck me—that even though we had been doing well for a year, there was a lot of room for improvement."

Hemmer, whose goal was to be in better shape by his 40th birthday than he was at his 30th, instantly saw results—in fat loss and in energy levels. "I noticed when I was going up the steps to a loading dock, I went up two steps at a time and I didn't even blink, and I realized I had never done that. I just felt lighter." After the first 2 weeks, Krista even made the comment that they had eaten better the past 2 weeks than they ever had before in their 12 years of marriage.

The rewards kept coming: Krista has lost 15 pounds and a dress size, Pete's down from a nearly 44-size pants to almost a 34, it's easier to take care of the kids, friends who haven't seen them in months don't even recognize them, and they're even planning a sea kayaking trip. "That wouldn't have happened before," Hemmer says. "For us, sitting on the sofa and watching a pay-per-view movie was the extent of our physical activity."

When he went to the gym to have his body composition checked after 6 weeks, the woman who ran the machine looked at Hemmer's 6-week improvement and asked him what he was doing. "I told her briefly about that the Abs Diet, and she said that even the gym's weight-loss program doesn't get such good results," Hemmer says. "She also said that it appeared that my body had become efficient at burning fat. I told her politely that it was sort of the whole point."

And, of course, there's also one other side effect: "Our sex life has improved dramatically," Pete says. "Krista says that if I get in any better shape, she's going to need smelling salts."

val workout per week to complement your strength training. Your mode of transportation isn't important, so pick whatever activity you prefer. What's important is making sure you change gears. You can vary it in whatever time frames you want (1-minute high-intensity, 1-minute low-intensity, or maybe build up with 30 seconds of high, rest, then 45 seconds, then rest, and so on). Always warm up and cool down for at least 5 minutes at the beginning and end of each interval workout.

Sample Workout Schedule

You'll do circuit training 3 days a week, making sure you have at least 1 day of rest in between days. Additionally, do an interval workout 1 day a week. You also have the option of doing light cardiovascular exercise (cycling, walking, swimming, tennis, or golf without the cart) on your off days. On these days, make having fun your main goal—don't think about calorie burns, afterburns, George Burns, or any other kind of burns.

Monday: Circuit Training
Tuesday (optional): Walking at brisk pace or light cardiovascular exercise
Wednesday: Circuit Training
Thursday (optional): Walking at brisk pace or light cardiovascular exercise
Friday: Circuit Training
Saturday: Interval Workout
Sunday: Off

The Abs Diet Workout Worksheet

Like naked bodies, all workouts are not made alike. If you're currently not exercising, then anything is better than a nightly chips festival on the love seat. But for the most powerful workouts for burning fat and adding muscle, follow the Abs Diet Workout Worksheet.

Your goal here is to amass a total of 40 points per week. For each activity, you get full credit for doing the activity continuously for 20 minutes. Exercises in the Abs Diet Workout give you the highest number of points, but if you can't keep to that workout schedule, you can sneak in a few extra points here and there to make your workout work. Don't try to go over 40 points a week, though—there's no extra credit for total exhaustion.

10 POINTS (FOR EACH 20 MINUTES SPENT)

Abs Diet Circuit	Interval Training (solo sport: running, swimming, cycling, or machine)
Abdominals Circuit	

6 POINTS (FOR EACH 30 MINUTES SPENT)

Abs-specific classes	Mountain biking, intermediate to advanced, hilly course
Basketball (full-court)	
Boot Camp classes	Pilates, advanced
Boxing	Power lifting
Bull running, Pamplona	Snowshoeing, hilly
Calisthenics: pushups, pullups, situps	Spinning classes
	Sports-conditioning classes
Cross-country skiing, hilly	Stairclimbing, stadium stairs
Hiking, hilly	Strength training, noncircuit
Hockey, inline or ice	Volleyball, beach, competitive

4 POINTS (FOR EACH 30 MINUTES SPENT)

Basketball, (half-court)	Downhill skiing, intermediate to advanced
BOSU classes	
Dodgeball	Kickboxing classes
Inline skating, steady	Martial arts

4 POINTS (FOR EACH 30 MINUTES SPENT) (CONT.)

Pilates, beginner	Strength-training, ultra-light weights
Racquetball	
Rowing machine, steady pace	Surfing
Rugby	Swimming, steady pace
Soccer	Tennis, competitive
Step classes	Ultimate Frisbee
Strength-training, resistance bands	Volleyball, indoor
	Yoga, advanced or power

3 POINTS (FOR EVERY 30 MINUTES SPENT)

Adventure racing	Kayaking/canoeing
Cross-country skiing, flat	Rock climbing
Cycling, road, steady pace, flat	Snowboarding
Dance-aerobic classes	Stairclimbing machine, steady pace
Downhill skiing, easy	Tennis, recreational
Fishing, big-league tuna	Urban Rebounding classes
Golf, without cart	Volleyball, beach, recreational
Hiking, flat	Walking, brisk
Jogging, steady pace	Yoga, beginner

2 POINTS (FOR EVERY 30 MINUTES SPENT)

Basketball, solo	Ice skating, recreational
Bowling	Softball
Fishing, recreational	Stretching, general
Frisbee golf	Walking, slow
Gardening	Water aerobics classes
Golf, driving range	Wrestling, with kids
Golf, with cart	Yoga, meditative

ABS DIET FAQ

How does the Abs Diet differ from other diets?

Following most popular diet books is like sending your body to prison—they're all about deprivation and restriction. These diets may work in the short term by shackling you to keep you away from certain foods and calories. But once you get a sniff of freedom (in the form of fries and shakes), you're more likely to try to escape. And you know the severe penalties for trying to escape—a life sentenced to a fat gut.

The Abs Diet is about gaining, not restricting. You gain a leaner, firmer body, more control over your life, and even more opportunities to enjoy the foods you love. By eating six times a day, you'll keep your energy levels high and your hunger always at bay, while training your body to burn calories and make itself lean. You'll feed yourself the foods that force your body to lose weight, to burn more calories.

What about really popular ones, like Atkins and South Beach?

The Atkins Diet eliminates practically all carbohydrates for the first part of the plan, leaving you with only foods that contain protein and fat. It's a gimmick that works—in the short term. By restricting the foods you eat to only a handful of them, you'll automatically drop pounds because you've dramatically reduced your total calories. But you'll also dramatically reduce your intake of vitamins, minerals, and fiber, while upping your intake of artery-clogging saturated fats. The one good thing about Atkins: It eliminates empty carb calories like doughnuts and Doritos. But on the Abs Diet, you dump the lousy carbs and keep the healthy and delicious ones (whole-grain bread, cereal, fruit, vegetables), which will keep you full, fuel your body, and dampen your cravings.

The South Beach Diet is based on sound principles of healthy nutrition, and it's a pretty good choice for pure weight loss. But the Abs Diet isn't just about losing weight—it's about turning unsightly flab into lean, sexy muscle. That's why, unlike South Beach, the Abs Diet features muscle-building exercise as part of its foundation. Muscle exponentially speeds up the fat-burning process—1 pound of muscle requires your body to burn up to 50 calories a day just to maintain that muscle. This plan combines exercise with the foods that most promote muscle growth.

There are many diets out there today, and as long as people have the opportunity to choose a course for better health, that's what ultimately counts. Frankly, I hate the word *diet,* because diet implies that you have to eliminate and restrict, but to call this the Abs Nutritional Superiority Plan seemed a bit much.

How much weight will I lose?

I can't give you a firm number, because people's bodies have more variables than a calculus textbook. I can tell you that some people who have used the Abs Diet have lost 25 pounds in 6 weeks. That doesn't necessarily mean that you will, but it means that you might or that you could. Much of your success depends on so many factors—including your intensity of exercise and your starting weight. But we've seen a lot of people who've lost somewhere between 10 and 15 pounds in the first 6 weeks while also gaining a few pounds of muscle, which helps them keep burning fat after that initial 6-week surge.

What percentage of body fat do you have to get to so that you can see your abs?

Finding your abs might feel as daunting as digging through sand to find a buried treasure. But if you dig diligently enough—and by that I mean burning off that extra, unwanted flab—you will find the treasure. As far as the specific body-fat percentage, it varies. I've seen both men and women with body-fat percentages in the teens with defined stomach muscles. For most men, you need to get to around 10 percent. The good news is that if you're exercising regularly, then at least 80 percent of every pound you lose will be fat.

Will it work for women?

Absolutely. It doesn't take a Peeping Tom to know that men and women have some distinct physiological differences, but in this case, what works for a man will also work for a woman. This eating plan revolves around eating foods that are good for everyone, and the exercise plan is about building lean muscle mass, not linebacker muscle mass. The key is not to count calories but to eat six meals a day to keep you properly fueled. A woman's portion sizes can be a little smaller than a man's, but by eating well-balanced meals with the ABS DIET POWER 12, anyone can lose fat.

So the ABS DIET POWER 12 foods are the only ones I can eat?

Absolutely not. You build your diet around the ABS DIET POWER 12—and make sure you have several of them at every meal and snack. You can supplement with other foods, but if your meals are centered on the Powerfoods, you'll ensure yourself a well-balanced diet that keeps you satiated and provides you with the ingredients that help keep your body properly fueled and turn it into a fat-burning machine.

What about portion control? Can I eat any amount I want?

If you're eating these Powerfoods, they should take care of your hunger so that you don't have the physical urge to eat a lot. By doing things like eating six times a day and making sure you get enough fiber, you'll decrease the chance of shoveling enormous amounts of food into your mouth. That said, it's always smart to be aware of how much you eat—especially when you're starting out. You can cover your plate with the ABS DIET POWER 12, but there's no need to pile the food so high that you need a city council permit to construct your plate. Let's just say that a height restriction is in effect.

The Abs Diet includes a weekly cheat meal. Does that mean I really can eat anything?

Yes. One time a week, you can eat anything. You want a Bavarian cream? Eat it. You want a plate of wings? Eat it. You want fried

---

ABS DIET SUCCESS STORY

HE INSPIRED HIS WIFE—AND HIS SON

Name: Bill and Kathy Bartz
Bill's age: 56
Height: 5'9"
Weight, Week 1: 187
Weight, Week 6: 170
Weight, Week 12: 166
Body-fat percentage, Week 1: 18.7
Body-fat percentage, Week 12: 10.2
Kathy's height: 5'6"
Weight, Week 1: 126
Weight, Week 12: 118

Last year, Bill Bartz made a New Year's resolution: He wanted to see his six-pack before the end of the year. He had been lifting weights regularly for 15 years, so he had a lot of bulky muscle mass, but he was missing the definition.

"I saw the author on *Good Morning America* on the Fourth of July, and I thought, hmmmmm," Bartz says. "So I decided to go to Border's and get the book. I just started reading it and it all made sense. And what I really liked was how it took other diets and blew them apart."

alligator? Eat it. The cheat meal is designed to reward you for good work throughout the week and help keep cravings in check. And what we found is that once people start seeing results, many don't even want the cheat meal—because the ABS DIET POWER 12 satisfy so many different kinds of cravings. The only caveat is that you must limit yourself to just one cheat meal a week. Do it any more, and you might as well be on the Doughnut Diet.

Can I make food substitutions for the ABS DIET POWER 12?

Many of the 12 categories are broad enough to include many different dietary choices. Low-fat dairy includes milk, yogurt,

So Bartz decided to jump on the Abs Diet, and the pounds jumped off.

"One day, as I was getting out of the shower with a towel wrapped around me, my wife said, 'Whoa, that thing is working.'" So Bartz's wife, Kathy, joined in, too. With not much weight to lose, Kathy went from 126 pounds to 118.

Bartz took ab-specific classes 3 days a week at the gym, continued lifting weights, and incorporated interval training into his workouts.

But maybe the best outcome of the program is what it's done for his overall health. He's taking part in a clinical study in which his blood pressure is measured every 6 months. Since he started, his BP dropped from 130/90 to around 115/70. "When I went there, they were blown away," he says. "Right away, they noticed a difference in weight and they noticed a drastic drop in blood pressure. The nurse even wanted the name of the book so she could get one for her husband."

Bartz has been spreading the word about the Abs Diet—now, he's in competition with his 25-year-old son in a race for the first one to get a six-pack. His son isn't on the Abs Diet—and he' s losing out. Bartz says, "Last Saturday, I sent him a picture and he said, 'Dad, that's not you. You found that picture on the Internet.'

"I'm not at a six-pack yet, but I'm darn close," Bartz says, "and I know I'll have that six-pack for the end of the year."

cheese, and lean meat can include turkey, beef, fish, and chicken, for example. We do offer some substitution examples for different kinds of foods. Even if you're allergic to one category of food— nuts, for example—you can still figure out what ingredient you're missing by not eating that food and make up for it somewhere else. So having avocado or pumpkin seeds can give you the monounsaturated fats found in nuts—without the danger of an allergic reaction. (That said, if you do suffer from food allergies, consult your doctor before trying this or any other diet plan.)

Some of the smoothie recipes have cooked instant oatmeal. That sounds gross. How does it taste?

Recipes are a little like CD collections—what works for me might not work for you. But from the smoothies I've had, I can't even taste the oatmeal after it's blended—especially when there are berries or chocolate whey powder in them. So be brave and give it a go: Oatmeal adds bulk to the smoothie as well as the all-important satiating fiber.

What about this issue of targeting body fat? I thought you couldn't spot-reduce.

Well, you can't spot-reduce per se. That's a myth. But when you lose weight on the Abs Diet—particularly if you're doing some moderate exercise at the same time—you'll lower your body fat and will likely notice much of that loss around your midsection, since that's where most of the fat accumulates. And if you are doing ab workouts and strengthening those muscles, then as the fat peels away, you'll begin to see the washboard.

MEASURING YOUR PROGRESS ON THE ABS DIET

EVERY PERSON HAS HIS or her own way of measuring success on a diet. Some measure it by the way their pants feel. Some measure it by the compliments they receive. Some measure it by the fact that they no longer have to buy two seats when they fly cross-country. But if you want harder numbers to know where you stand, here are some pretty good ways to gauge your progress.

Weight. Pounds lost help give you some idea, but it's an incomplete number because it doesn't take into account the amount of muscle you're going to develop over the course of a plan. Muscle weighs more than fat, so even a dramatic fat loss may not translate into a dramatic drop in body weight.

Body mass index. The BMI is a formula that takes into consideration your height and your weight, and gives you an indication of whether you're overweight, obese, or in good shape. To calculate your BMI, the easiest thing to do is use an online calculator, like the one at MensHealth.com/BMI. A BMI between 25 and 30 indicates that you're overweight. Over 30 signifies obesity. BMI has its flaws as well (it doesn't take into account muscle mass, and it also leaves out another important factor—weight distribution, i.e. where most of the fat on your body resides). But for most people, it's a better indicator of progress than simply body weight itself.

Waist-to-hip ratio. Researchers have recently started using waist size and its relationship to hip size as a more definitive way to determine your health risk. It's considered more important than BMI because visceral fat—the fat that pushes your waist out in front of you—is a leading indicator for diabetes and heart disease. British researchers recently reported that men with waists of 40 or more inches, and women with waists of 35 or more, are at substantially higher risk for these diseases—up to four times higher.

That's why I want you to concentrate on lowering your waist-to-hip ratio. To figure out yours, measure your waist at your belly

ABS DIET SUCCESS STORY

A FORMER KICKBOXER KICKS IT INTO GEAR

Name: Ray and Kim Welborn

Ray's age: 44

Height: 5'8"

Weight, week 1: 188

Weight, week 6: 169

When he was in his twenties, Ray Welborn weighed in at about 130 pounds—it was his fighting weight as a professional kickboxer. But after he stopped, he started putting on the pounds. One day recently, he and his wife, Kim, were in the bookstore and saw the *Abs Diet*. They immediately took to it—Ray for what he thought it could do for his body, and Kim because it reminded her of the way her parents brought her up to eat healthy.

Ray, who's lost nearly 20 pounds, and Kim, who's lost 7, follow the weekly meal planner in the original Abs Diet. "That's our bible," Ray says. "And we stick to it. We even find that we can't eat as much on our cheat meal because of our shrinking bellies."

button and your hips at the widest point (around your butt). Divide your waist by your hips. For example, if your hips measure 40 inches and your waist at belly-button level measures 38 inches, your waist-to-hip ratio is 0.95. You want a waist-to-hip ratio of 0.92 or lower.

Body-fat percentage. Though this is the most difficult for the average person to measure because it requires a bit of technology, it's the most useful. That's because it doesn't just take into consideration weight, but also how much of your weight is fat and how much is muscle. Many gyms offer body-fat measurements, or you can try an at-home body-fat calculator. If you want a simple

---

With the meals, they adjusted recipes just a bit—so that Kim would eat ⅘ of a portion. That's when she started seeing a change. "I like it because of the healthy food," Kim says. "I used to do Weight Watchers, and they all concentrated just on points—it didn't matter whether it had high-fructose corn syrup in it or not. With Weight Watchers, I was always hungry. With this, I'm never hungry."

Both Ray and Kim have lost the weight from their bellies, and Ray is seeing muscles he hasn't seen in years, including ones right around his rib cage. "She really feels it when she cuddles up to me," he says.

More importantly, Ray *feels* healthier. "I feel lighter. My knees don't hurt as much anymore. With the excess weight off, it doesn't hurt to go downstairs like it used to," he says. "And I can tell you. I can bend over and tie my shoes and breathe at the same time. Seriously."

low-tech test (and this isn't as accurate as what the electronic versions will give you), try this: Sit in a chair with your knees and your feet flat on the floor. Using your thumb and index finger, gently pinch the skin on top of your right thigh. Measure the thickness of the pinched skin with a ruler. If it's ¾ inch or less, you have about 14 percent body fat—ideal for a guy, quite fit for a woman. If it's an inch, you're probably closer to 18 percent fat, which is a tad high for a man, but desirable for a woman. If you pinch more than an inch, you're at increased risk for diabetes and heart disease.

This last measurement can be the most significant because it'll really help give you a sense of how well you're sticking to a plan. As you see your body-fat percentage decrease, you'll see an increase in the amount of visible muscle. Experts say that in order for your abs to show, your body fat needs to be between 7 and 10 percent. For the average slightly overweight man, that means cutting body fat in about half. If you want to see your progress, take measurements every 2 weeks or so—and certainly not every day.

MEASUREMENT	START	END OF WEEK 2	END OF WEEK 4	END OF WEEK 6
Weight				
BMI				
Waist-to-hip ratio				
Body-fat percentage*				

Make sure to have the same person administer body-fat readings using the same method to ensure consistency.

INDEX

Underscored page references indicate sidebars and charts. **Boldface** references indicate illustrations.

NOTES

NOTES

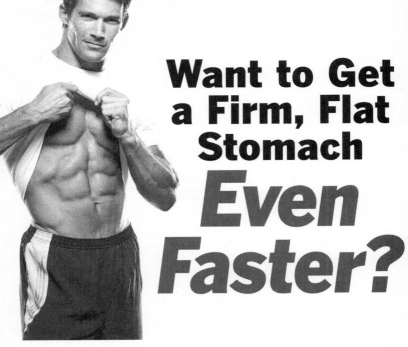